In Sickness
and in Play

The Rutgers Series
in Childhood Studies

Edited by
Myra Bluebond-Langner

Advisory Board
Joan Jacob Brumberg
Perri Kass
Jill Korbin
Bambi Schieffelin
Enid Schildkraut

In Sickness and in Play

CHILDREN COPING WITH CHRONIC ILLNESS

Cindy Dell Clark

Rutgers University Press
NEW BRUNSWICK, NEW JERSEY, LONDON

Library of Congress Cataloging-in-Publication Data

Clark, Cindy Dell.
  In sickness and in play : children coping with chronic illness /
Cindy Dell Clark.
      p. cm. — (Series in childhood studies)
      Includes bibliographical references and index.
      ISBN 0-8135-3269-8 (cloth : alk. paper) — ISBN 0-8135-3270-1 (pbk. :
alk. paper)
      1. Asthma in children—Psychological aspects—Case studies.
   2. Diabetes in children—Psychological aspects—Case studies.
   3. Adjustment (Psychology) in children.   I. Title.   II. Series.
      RJ436.A8 C535   2003
      618.92—dc21   2002015871

British Cataloging-in-Publication data for this book is available from the
British Library

The publication program of Rutgers University Press is supported by the
Board of Governors of Rutgers, The State University of New Jersey.

Manufactured in the United States of America

In tribute to the memory of Roger John Dell

Contents

Acknowledgments

In a scene from Jane Wagner's comic play *Search for Signs of Intelligent Life in the Universe,* a vulgar streetwalker being interviewed by a reporter stakes a claim to authorship of the reporter's written story.[1] The reporter only wrote down the narrative of her life, she taunted, while she herself *lived* it.

I have witnessed and interpreted that which patients and parents have *lived* with considerable fortitude and courage. Children and parents came to trust me over the course of my visits to their homes, and to entrust me with painful memories about chronic illness, as well as with play and friendship. To these generous informants, I owe a debt beyond reckoning. Although the identities of the parents and children have been disguised in the text out of concern for privacy, these families' due share of my writings I humbly concede.

I am also grateful to Holly Blackford, Melissa Gerdes, and Kathy Sullivan, who served as participant-observers and staff members at summer camps for chronically ill children. These researchers took on a demanding assignment with responsibility to the children's needs, as well as to the research. Each of these researcher-caretakers did impressive double duty.

I am thankful to several other organizations and individuals for aiding this investigation. First, there are the sponsoring organizations of the three summer camps, which remain anonymous to protect the privacy of the campers. Second, Focuscope Unlimited recruited family participants for the in-home research with painstaking accuracy and follow-through. Third, DePaul University's Kellstadt Center provided welcome funding for the pilot research. Fourth, the Rainbow Foundation for Children's Research and its donors covered expenses for the remaining fieldwork. Finally, the University of Pennsylvania provided me with institutional support through a visiting faculty arrangement that allowed me resources to finish much of the secondary research and writing. Paul Rozin was instrumental in arranging this privilege, for which I stand thankful.

Linda Alwitt, Holly Blackford, Elizabeth Monroe-Cook, Debra Stephens, Cathy Sweitzer, Gene Myers, Peggy Miller, Sue O'Curry, and Robert Pitts in various ways encouraged or sustained me through the wrenching process of entering (in fieldwork) the decidedly uncarefree world of childhood asthma and diabetes. Reactions to analytical work in progress were provided by many of these same colleagues, as well as by Joe DeRivera, Carl Johnson, Karl Rosengren, Jack Santino, and Ted Sarbin. Particular appreciation also goes to Myra Bluebond-Langer, whose work pointed the way and established the path for medical anthropology among children, and who has supported my work in countless ways. The able librarians at Penn State patiently helped me during the last phases of research, and indeed, Sara Whilden came up with the title for this book. Never underestimate the power of a great librarian. I want to thank my physician, David Prince, for being a model practitioner, and for serving as a technical consultant on the asthma background information. Jonathan Monroe-Cook helped with input on the interview material that only an insightful young person could provide. Lastly, my thanks go to Bill Clark, for lovingly supporting this labor of love during all the arduous phases of research and book writing.

I have witnessed childhood asthma firsthand, having grown up the sister of a brother with severe asthma. My late brother, Roger Dell, lived life with considerable gusto, despite the fearsome hazards of his breathless wheezing and unwelcome afflictions.

This book is dedicated to his memory and irrepressible spirit—
with the dream that juvenile chronic illness will rest more lightly
on future children. I believe that a crucial step toward improving
children's plight is within our reach, if we try to better grasp children's experiences from their own perspective.

CHAPTER 1

Introduction

Know you what it is to be a child? . . . It is to have a spirit still
streaming from the waters of baptism; . . . it is to turn
pumpkins into coaches and mice into horses, lowness into
loftiness, and nothing into everything, for each child has its
fairy godmother in its soul.   SHELLEY

Reality is something you rise above.   LIZA MINNELLI

*T*oday's fairy-tale ethos of American childhood, according to
which children are meant to live happily ever after, not to die too
soon, reckons poorly with serious childhood illness. The notion of
a child dying makes a discernible bump on the cultural Richter
scale, putting off-kilter our sense of things, unbalancing the scales
of justice. Health care, in our culture, is meant to banish death until its due hour at a ripe old age, if it must arrive at all. Children are
to be protected, and we are sickened when they are not.[1]

Child-serving charities, such as the Make-A-Wish Foundation and its many compatriots, are prone to redress terminal disease through means of altered reality—by gifting young patients
with a "wish come true" during their remaining months of life.
Wishes might involve visiting Disney World, or meeting a famous
athlete, a movie star, or the president, as well as (in one case I know)
breaking the world's record for the number of get-well cards received. Adults, who have survived longer yet so often live life less
intensely than do children, face an existential dilemma when confronting fatal childhood illness.[2] When life can end so soon, in a
manner so morally unjustified, we mature beings are made to grap-
ple with our own tenuous aliveness. If children can be cut down by
death, so can any one of us. In the face of an ill child, we somehow

want to rebalance the scales. Granting the last wishes of a child is a last resort to subvert death's insinuations.

But what about the child who carries a lasting, medically treatable chronic condition, an illness a child must learn to live with rather than die from? This child, of course, also deserves attention and compassion. Diabetes and severe asthma, the two examples dealt with in this book, involve daily treatments, pervasive adjustments in lifestyle, spells of physical suffering, and symbolic threats to essential life needs (that is, breath or nourishment). Fears and indignities lurk and seep into the childhoods of those with asthma or diabetes, spreading unhappily over the ordinary routines of upbringing. Chronic illness, as will be documented in this book, affects many, many children.[3] Children with chronic illness, according to numerous studies, are at greater risk than others of developing mental health or social adjustment problems.[4] And the impact of childhood chronic illness is not diminishing. Asthma, a particularly prevalent childhood disorder, has been gaining ground in both incidence and fatality in recent years.[5]

As this book will chronicle, the reality of chronic illness can be harrowing both for children and for their families. Yet there is also heartening news. The challenge of chronic illness is one that families can and regularly do rise to meet. The ordeal can be surmounted, partly because children have impressive capacities to imagine and transcend what cannot be cured. A young girl might fancy that her blood-check device used in the treatment of diabetes represents a blood-sucking polar bear with a prickly "kiss." A boy with diabetes might fantasize that the insulin-filled syringe, with its lines of demarcation, is a zebra. Children do not need Mary Poppins's wizardry to make the medicine go down, for they cast their own spells on illness to make the suffering and treatment more bearable. Children use pretend play, story, ritual, and humor, as well as trusted playthings, to work for themselves the kind of "nursery magic" by which the fictional Velveteen Rabbit soothed illness. Children serve as their own shamanic healers, as the ultimate child-life specialists, through the phenomenon of imaginal coping.

The explorations I recount in this book were conducted in the homes and summer camps of young children with severe asthma or diabetes, in their own social domains, where they could give voice to their own ways of experiencing chronic illness.[6] Diabetes and severe asthma, illnesses requiring in-home treatment outside the clinical or hospital setting, comprised my subject. I was attracted to studying these illnesses because they significantly affect the lives of children at home more than at the hospital. Past research on children's illness mainly has used a hospital or clinic setting, each a cultural location that foregrounds or emphasizes the biomedical treatment process and affords children little privacy.[7] Teaching hospitals, in particular, have been accessible sites for much research among children. Yet teaching hospitals are apt to be outstanding, rather than typical or representative, in their treatment of a child's medical needs and often have available the services of a child-life worker who addresses the child's total needs, including emotional distress.[8]

My project was grassroots based, carried out in forty-six urban and suburban homes of diverse social class and ethnicity in the Chicago metropolitan area during the mid-1990s. (For a detailed description of study method and design, see Appendix A.) Most of the children studied were ages five to eight years. Some children were fortunate to receive treatment from highly trained medical specialists, who in exceptional cases addressed the child's emotional, social, and medical needs in the program of treatment. More typically, a child's care was not oriented toward treating the "whole child" and was not entirely state-of-the-art even in its medical regimen, particularly for asthma. For example, many young study participants with asthma did not recognize and had never used a peak-flow meter, a gauge of breathing function that was largely standard issue in elite medical institutions in the mid-1990s.[9]

I did not focus on judging the value of medical treatment; my purpose was to open a window into the felt human experience of symptoms, suffering, and treatment encountered by a cross-section of young children, understood from their own vantage point. My goal was to witness the lived experience of illness within the lifeworld of children. I sought to bring to the fore children's perceptions, feelings, and understandings as they lived with chronic illness. I also listened to their parental caretakers, for illness takes hold in families, as well.

The child-centered approach shed light on both the positive and negative sides of the chronic illness among youngsters. Children's worlds included not only significant felt suffering, but also creative, resilient ways of rising above the hardship and stress, often through imaginative means. The children showed that burdens are often counterbalanced by the power of narrative and fantasy. This book attempts to address both the depths and heights of children's experiences, both the magnitude of their dilemma and their resourceful "imaginal coping."

In Chapters 2 and 3, the experience of diabetes and asthma are presented to provide a context for understanding children's illness experiences. The context for each illness necessarily touches on sociocultural issues as well as concerns of the family and individual. Children's overall propensity to cope through imagination, as well as their coping through humor and ritual, is the topic of Chapter 4. Chapter 5 will raise some final themes, including the issue of how imaginal coping taps into a lifeline of cultural symbols, using them for healing.

To attain medical care to their liking, a significant portion of American adults have come to embrace (and in some cultural traditions have long practiced) non-allopathic, alternative forms of treatment for illness.[10] One basis for the alternative health care movement has been a desire for health care to have a broader framework of meaning, extending to psychological and social dimensions as well as the physical body.[11] Ritual and symbolic behaviors such as visualization or prayer are features that accompany the practices of alternative healing. The alternative medicine movement views the patient as having wrongly been treated as "childlike" in conventional biomedicine rather than receiving the respect due adults as partners in the medical process.

This study of very young patients demonstrates that the literally childlike have much to teach about the value of symbolism and ritual, as well as the value of respecting the patient's full humanity. Lacking any organized social movement (albeit summer camp qualifies as a shared social experience), children addressed issues of emotion and meaning through their personal resources of imagination and trust. Children's own voices, about their own illness experience, contain an enlightening measure of insight— perhaps insight that can tip the unbalanced scales of childhood chronic illness. Adults need only to bravely and respectfully listen.

CHAPTER 2

Juvenile Diabetes

Insulin-dependent diabetes mellitus (IDDM or Type 1) defines a group of patients who are literally dependent on exogenous insulin to prevent ketoacidosis and death. This type of diabetes is associated with certain histocompatibility antigens (HLA) on chromosome six, with autoimmunity directed against the islet.   MERCK MANUAL, 1987

Diabetes means you always get hurt. It's boring. You have to put your finger on the machine.

FIVE-YEAR-OLD BOY WITH DIABETES

Scientific understanding of diabetes as a biomedical entity and the treatment marvels thereby possible have enabled children with the illness to survive and grow into adulthood. But make no mistake: The admirable technical "fix" has not eradicated children's suffering. A nine-year-old I interviewed, who was diagnosed with type 1 diabetes at age six, knew this well. She had pricked her finger for a blood test nine thousand times and received more than two thousand insulin shots in the past three years. She typically has four blood checks a day, eats on a relentlessly regular schedule, and may wake up out-of-kilter at night when her blood-sugar level drops.[1] The "adjustments" necessitated by diabetes—which as far as she knows will be lifelong—are wrenching.

This chapter will describe how the medical treatment for diabetes presents young patients and their families with unique trials at a tender age. Before proceeding, however, some medical briefing on diabetes is in order, to provide a description of children's medical treatment and its biomedical rationale.

Diabetes

The American Diabetes Association has described insulin-dependent diabetes as follows: "Insulin-dependent (type 1) diabetes refers to a complete or near-complete inability of the body to make insulin. To survive, people with this type of diabetes depend on daily injections of insulin. . . . The vast majority of children with diabetes have the insulin-dependent type. . . . The person with insulin-dependent diabetes can have wide daily swings in blood-sugar levels." [2]

The daily swings in blood-sugar levels can encompass two acute complications, in a medical sense. At one end of the spectrum is the possibility of being "high" in blood sugar (hyperglycemia), and in turn high in levels of ketoacids in the blood. This condition of severely high blood sugar can lead to coma or death. At the other end of a not-very-pleasant spectrum is the possibility of "low" blood sugar (hypoglycemia or insulin reaction), which can result when insulin lowers the blood-sugar level too severely. Low blood sugar can lead to loss of consciousness or to seizures, if untreated. The experience of a low reaction, characterized by such symptoms as shakiness, confusion, headache, or irritability, can have a rapid onset.

Periodic checks of blood-sugar levels via a finger poke and a portable blood-glucose monitor aid in adjusting a child's insulin level to avoid these dangerous extremes. Amounts of insulin given are balanced against carefully monitored blood-glucose readings, food intake, and exercise levels. Children typically receive two, or sometimes three, injections of insulin over the course of a day, with blood checks taken even more frequently so that insulin can be properly dosed. In a nondiabetic person, by contrast, the pancreas automatically and naturally adjusts the amount of insulin secreted to balance with exercise and eating, a homeostatic process that must be mimicked by human action in the case of type 1 diabetes.

Medical experts emphasize that maintaining blood-sugar levels as close to normal as possible can delay or prevent the long-term complications that can affect diabetic individuals many years after onset.[3] Complications of juvenile diabetes during adulthood can include kidney disease, heart disease, and damage to the blood vessels in the eye, potentially leading to blindness. Thus, there are both short-term and long-term health-related incentives for maintaining good control.

Derived from Western biomedicine, the explanatory model for type 1 diabetes (as just described, involving insulin and blood-sugar levels) is only one way to represent diabetes. Allopathic physicians are trained to think of diabetes as a biomedical entity, as a disease constituted at a formal, abstract level, understandable apart from human experience.[4] Yet diabetes as a human matter exists in context: in an individual patient, of a particular cultural and social milieu, in a particular family, at a certain age.[5] Although most contemporary American adults place great trust in biomedical discourse and its practices, the felt world of youngsters introduces a quite different definition for diabetes, and another frame of reference that predominates for the child.[6]

Diabetes in a Child's Lifeworld

To better convey the lively and interactive flavor of the illness experience, this chapter and the next use the rhetorical device of first-person commentaries. These commentaries set forth the views and experiences of children juxtaposed with the views and experiences of adult caregivers, representing the distinctive renderings of illness by children versus adults. The fragments of discourse assembled in the commentaries draw from interview material, parent journals, and records which were mined, recombined, or reworded for the sake of coherence. The commentaries differ from speech that appears in quotation marks, which represents verbatim utterances from individual respondents. Throughout, the edited commentaries are true to the original tone and intent of informants and represent recurrent themes of concern to children and adults. While the commentaries are meant to be vivid portrayals—mosaics or collages of edited discourse—they carry the weight of authority, having been carefully derived from patterns of response across numerous families.[7]

It's Saturday morning, and Mom woke me up early to eat breakfast, take a blood test, and get a shot. It's that way every day, even when there's no school. Sometimes Mom lets me go back to bed afterwards, but I always have to get up first to eat and get tested and get a shot. I sit at the kitchen table, eating cereal and juice. I have to eat cereal that comes without sugar, but sometimes my mom lets me put a few pieces of sugar cereal on top. The doorbell is ringing. I think my mom is getting it. It is Cindy. She wants to interview me about what it's like to have diabetes. She has a big case full of toys and things for drawing and pictures to look at. She lets me dump out some toys. This might be fun, playing with her. She has a doctor's kit with toy shots and medical things, and dolls to use with the shots and things. She has little toys of a hospital bed and people from the hospital, and even a teddy bear small enough to play with at the hospital. I have toys of my own just the same size, from my dollhouse. Can we play with both our toys together? She says yes. So I run off to get my toys. My mom calls me, though, before I can get them. She's always doing this, interrupting fun.

Go in the kitchen and finish your breakfast! Half your cereal is still in the bowl and you need to finish your juice, too.

The procedures involved in treating diabetes permeate a child's lifeworld. Childhood play is punctuated by interruptions to stop, shift attention, and check blood, eat a snack, finish a meal, or get a shot. In field notebooks and when talking with me, mothers recorded how fun activities had to be cut short to allow for scheduled treatment. "I think it's . . . an inconvenience, that you have to test now," said one mother. "They're swimming in the pool, and you have to test." Upon interruptions of fun, parents reported that children would poignantly protest, "I wish I didn't have diabetes."

Even on occasions that might be carefree for other children, diabetic children (and their caretakers) can never leave cares behind. Blood checks must be done even at the circus, if the schedule dictates. Sleepover parties require arrangements for a blood test and shot. The school day includes a scheduled intrusion to use the blood-glucose monitor, eat a snack, or both, at a time announced by the teacher or by a wristwatch with a preset alarm.

Even vacations, intended to be a break from routine, involve intricate parental precautions to make sure that eating stays on schedule, that insulin is stored at the proper temperature and ready, and that other supplies are always available to treat lows or to test blood. The routine relentlessly intrudes without respite, even during time set aside for a relaxed family getaway. The orderliness of scheduled daily life can never be forgotten.

Treatment periodically invades, however briefly, a child's emotional and social space. Children spoke of being "poked" and "pricked" during blood tests, explaining that they were bothered or irritated at the regular intrusion into relaxed amusements, even if by fiat of medical necessity. Play must yield to the business of diabetes care, as the latter commands an unremitting right of way for attention.

When I asked children ages five to eight to define diabetes, most focused on *treatment* practices as the defining element—reflecting that this is the salient daily basis for encountering diabetes. Unseen bodily systems or abstract notions of glucose metabolism are outside the usual frame of reference for a young child. The child's definition instead reflects ordinary, day-to-day activities.

What is diabetes? "I don't know, it's just you get shots all the time" (boy, eight). "It's a disease that means you can't eat sugar" (girl, seven). "It's where you get shots, and you do blood in your finger" (girl, seven). "It's just you can't have much sugar, and you have to do blood tests and shots" (boy, seven).

Treatment procedures were an ever-present theme of conversations and play sessions with children. A child might use lay terminology, referring to a finger-sticking lancet used to check blood as a "pin" or "poker," but the treatment procedures and diet restrictions were all too familiar. Conversant about how to use syringes and the strips used in blood-glucose testing, children were experts in their own treatment.

> CDC: If you were going to meet somebody that never heard of diabetes, and they wanted to know what it's like for you to have it, what would you tell them?
> BOY (age eight): Uh, how to fill the insulin, how to do the blood test, how to clean the machine when you're finished. . . . How do you buy the pin? Where do you get the strips? . . . How much units you put in the number that you are in the book [referring to a book with recorded numerical readings from the blood-glucose monitor, and corresponding numerical "units" of insulin to be given].
> CDC: Lets say an alien landed here from another planet . . . and they said to you [Adopts mock voice of alien], "On my planet we don't have diabetes. Tell me what it's like to have diabetes?" What would you tell them?
> BOY (age seven): Um, you would have to get shots all the time . . . you would have to get blood tests. . . . You would have to eat stuff without sugar.
> CDC: What stuff could they eat? Like could they eat vegetables?

BOY: Mm hm [Nods agreement].

CDC: What couldn't they eat?

BOY: Pop Tarts.

CDC: No Pop Tarts for the alien if they have diabetes. Anything else?

BOY: Hmm, gummy sharks [candy].

CDC: No gummy sharks for the alien either.

As a way to probe children's feelings about diabetes, young informants were asked to sort through photos of varied settings—ranging from a lush green woods to a flooded river plain to a sunny playground—and select pictures that, to the child, had a "feeling" reminiscent of diabetes. (This Metaphor Sort Technique, or MST, is discussed in more detail in Appendix A.) One six-year-old girl chose a picture of a sunny playground, yet in explaining how this picture had a "diabetes feeling," she inserted an additional element. At the edge of the playground, she pointed out, there was a fence (not literally shown in the picture she chose) that "keeps you in"—within the playground's confines. Through this imagined visual metaphor, the child expressed boundaries that restricted the free range of playful experience—the figurative fence around the playground. The imagined fence, surrounding and containing the otherwise "happy" picture, made it (according to her) "sad" and "happy" at the same time. By describing the feeling of diabetes this way, she revealed it to be to be a part of her everyday life, tangential to pleasure but nevertheless restrictive.

While not all children imagined fences around the playground in just this way, most did describe a blend of positive and negative feelings associated with diabetes. Diabetes can involve "people who are nice to you" or can be pleasantly reminiscent of "being with your mom," who helps you; yet children had mixed feelings overall due to the necessity to endure shots or other hardships of treatment.

Parent as "Remote-Control Pancreas"

My dad is in a race today, and we are at the park where he's racing. Just look at this big slide. Isn't it so fun? And those are really good swings that swing really high. Come on, I'll show you. You can push us on the swing. My friend and I are running and playing, it's fun here. Come on. Have fun with us!

You don't look so good to me, dear. I have glucose tablets right here in my coat pocket. Take some. I can tell you're low. You've been running around and now you're low. Take some, come on. No more running around for now.

In the United States, biomedically oriented treatment often assumes a taken-for-granted cultural position of privilege. In turn it is assumed that biomedical treatment is a benign, desirable activity.[8] Problems that arise in treatment (resistance, forgetting, behavioral anomalies, etc.) tend to be regarded as a patient's inability to cope, as a problem in "compliance." Medical parlance views concerns over treatment as a regrettable trait of the "noncompliant" family or child.[9]

Yet as I have come to know the families of diabetic children in a home setting, my impression is that these families cooperate with a demanding medical routine with admirable constancy. In contexts ranging from playgrounds to campgrounds, and from school to pool, families steadfastly followed their regimen as if by second nature. Mothers, who were usually the main caretakers, made decisions about meals and snacks with the smooth habit of experience, as if these decisions were as effortless as knowing what coat or sweater to wear for particular weather. Over time, I came to realize that each mother (and now and then, a father) served as a kind of "remote-control pancreas"—a label that parents acknowledged as fitting. The parent caretaker monitored and took into account everything the child did and then dispensed food or insulin accordingly. It was common for the vigilant parent to notice when a child seemed "low," and to intervene to stave off a crisis. Children occasionally bemoaned the ubiquitous interventions, but by and large they cooperated.

So impressive was the disciplined habit of monitoring and calibrating childhood diabetes and treatment that it raises the inverse question of that posed by "compliance" researchers. That is, rather than searching out the roots of nonadherence, the inverse question should be asked. What accounts for the impressive degree of discipline and follow-through possible within families of diabetic children? How did the routine come to be so habitual? The answer traces partly to the social treatment of the onset of childhood diabetes, which serves, it appears, to fundamentally and effectively transform the family of the diagnosed child.

Becoming Diabetic: A Family Rite of Passage

When I first got diabetes, I had to go to the hospital. It was sad because I missed my friends, and I missed home. I had to lay in bed. I kept hearing someone cry, like there was a baby crying. So then I knew I wasn't the only person there. We got to go for short walks to the playroom and there were more kids there. They had video games, too, in the playroom. I felt better when I knew someone else was getting needles and shots done to them, not just me. The video games were fun to play.

I slept in her room at the hospital, because she was scared and didn't want me to leave. I kept thinking, her health depends on me. Will I be able to do this? The shots, the diet, everything else. I just kept thinking, her health depends on me. I was in shock, probably. And they're teaching me to draw up insulin, and inject it in an orange, and into her. And I'm thinking, her health depends on me.

Among the young informants who participated in this study, some were diagnosed as diabetic in infancy. As far back as the children could consciously recall, their daily experience had always been a matter of blood tests, shots, and time-structured diet control. Other children, diagnosed at a later age, vividly remembered their diagnosis and initial hospitalization, well enough to make drawings of it. Some re-created the hospital experience in playing with toy props (a miniature hospital bed, IV-stand, and figures of doctors, nurses, and medical implements). When all is said and done, however, the narrative of the initial onset of diabetic symptoms and the resulting hospitalization was clearly not the child's exclusive story. The tale had become a shared family narrative, a part of the family's commonly held lore, a story told around the child as well as by the child. The story was co-constructed, arising within the shared discourse of the child and her family.[10]

Parents' memories about the onset of their child's diabetes placed hospitalization in the foreground, when the child was medically stabilized and initial treatment planned. During this hospital stay, parents underwent rites tantamount to initiation: learning to dose insulin, to give shots, to plan the diet, to record blood tests, to recognize and treat insulin reactions (lows), and so on. Parental training in the principles and skills required to care for a diabetic child was both a looming necessity and an inescapable mandate. The learning process was intense, both in terms of mastering knowledge and mastering the concomitant feelings about the new activities. Emotional turmoil and grief typified the "period of adjustment." The parent faced a harsh transformation during a child's hospital stay. Comfortable assumptions had to be discarded and remade. Expected experience had to be refocused and reframed. Even families with a professional affiliation in health care who until now had been able to go home and abandon patient-care concerns at the end of the day found the adjustment jolting.

In the Peters family, for example, the oldest child, Patty (six years old upon being interviewed and the daughter of a dentist and a nurse), had been diagnosed at age twenty-two months. Mrs. Peters admitted that her prior "knowledge base for diabetes" as a nurse was "on the surface." "You don't see the twenty-four-hour workings, the day after day" of diabetes while working as a nurse, she explained. Having a child with diabetes had transformed her dentist husband as well. Formerly a "real heavy sleeper," Dr. Peters now wakes easily: "If I just call his name, he's standing straight up." Such is the twenty-four-hour state of alert required of a parent of a diabetic child.

Dr. Peters confirmed that his life priorities had been recast based on his daughter's diagnosis and hospitalization. "Before Patty became sick, I had an image of how life should be, and how my kids should be, and how perfect it should be." His post-diagnosis world was more open to compromise, in that life is "never quite what you expect it to be, and what you plan it to be, but that's okay, that's life." He no longer cared whether he was a "millionaire by age forty." He asserted that monetary or career concerns were now less important than "spending time with my kids."

A perceptible, irreversible shift in the parental universe grew out of each child's diabetic diagnosis and hospitalization. A shift in the way tasks are prioritized marked the end of the status quo for Mrs. Curtis, who sheepishly marveled that, before taking her son to the hospital, she had put a money-related errand ahead of his urgent need for care. Such miscalculations would no longer take place in her post-diagnosis mothering: "In the middle of the night I woke him up because I was concerned about him. . . . The first thing in the morning I went to the doctor's office." Her voice swells with emotion as she continues. "She [the doctor] said he's dehydrated. I'm going to do a blood test. . . . She caught [the diabetes] right away." Later that day, Mrs. Curtis said, she was on the phone with my sister. . . . I have to get this check to the bank. . . . I went to the bank before I took Tommy to the hospital. His sugar was only like 469 at the hospital, which is not bad. He's been that since then. . . . I have to laugh now because when I went to the bank, I had this check. . . . I didn't fill out the deposit slip and I put it in the [drive-through] teller. . . . I'm like "I've got a sick kid here, I'm sorry." . . . When I think back about it I think I can't believe I took this child to the bank instead of just going right to the hospital. . . . Why did I have to get to this bank? I guess I do know better now, too. . . . I can't believe I did that. Let's face it. The most important thing was getting him to the hospital.

The stated purpose of parent training at the hospital was to produce a proficient parent caretaker by teaching the practices and skills needed. But as Jean Lave and collaborators have documented in nonmedical domains, learning involves more than acquiring factual knowledge; it also conveys entry into a world of social practices.[11] Learning engenders changes in the whole person, in that the apprenticeship has a transforming impact on notions of reality and self as well as on cognitive skills. Put another way, the activity of learning is not just goal oriented (that is, oriented toward learning techniques of treatment), not just a matter of cognitive knowledge transfer, but it also constitutes a way of being, in the broadest sense.

As an example of how learning brings about a transformation of self, consider a related example: how medical students learn to engage and formulate reality biomedically through the practice of taking medical histories.[12] Taking a medical history is a learned interpretive act that formulates the patient's story not in terms of life experience, but in terms of a medical problem framed as a disease process. Learning to take and record the case history is a practice that transforms the students learning it, since the case history in effect serves to objectify or depersonalize the patient and at the same time to emotionally distance the doctor from the patient.[13] Becoming proficient in the case history method changes the social and affective orientation of the newly trained physician, over and above the build-up of skill and knowledge. The learning experience involves a transformation of self, with regard to how the physician encounters and makes sense of patients. The new knowledge constrains certain ways of being, such as empathy or emotional recognition, and expands other modes of being, including detached authority and control.[14]

Parents whose children are hospitalized upon diagnosis of diabetes likewise undergo transformations of self in the course of being indoctrinated to skills and facts. A new role identity (as a parent of a child with paramount, round-the-clock medical needs) is constructed along with the requisite technical training. That is, parents not only learn skills of giving shots, dispensing proper food, and treating or preventing highs and lows but also appear to embody and accept a pronounced change in the world as they know it. The parent now occupies a new reality: serving as the override manual pilot as surrogate for the child's pancreas (since the automatic pilot of the pancreas is not functional).

No wonder, then, that one mother referred to her weekend prior to the child's diagnosis and hospital stay as her "last normal weekend," since so much about her life and ways of seeing the world were transformed afterward. Another mother, whose second diabetic child did not benefit from such a hospitalization, found diagnosis *without* hospitalization to be almost too "normal," for the child as well as the parent: "There was no sense putting her in the hospital since we already know what to do. [With my first daughter] everybody had time to acclimate. I think [the hospitalization] . . . set it apart. . . . I feel kind of bad in that respect [for my other daughter] because it was like one day [suddenly] she had it. One day she didn't, and the next day she was like her [diabetic] sister. She didn't have that little period where she could adjust."

Just as a rite of passage provides a context in which the ritual participant becomes suspended between roles (neither still in the prior role, nor yet in the role-to-be), the hospital provided a kind of half-way house for the family grasping and accepting their child's diabetes.[15] Having a child in the hospital signaled "crisis" to the family's entire social network, so that extended family members mobilized their support by sending gifts, making visits, and now and then wanting to learn more about diabetes. Business-as-usual was interrupted, as the culturally meaningful setting of the hospital dictated. Meanwhile, parents felt they had a chance to adjust in the supportive environment of the hospital, since they were not yet solely responsible for their child's care. Indeed, the act of leaving the hospital was difficult for some parents, since it marked the final entry into their new role and assumptions. Having accepted a world in which "your child's health totally depends on you," parents had also accepted a reframed reality in which their role was continually, gravely important.

In contemporary U.S. society, babies usually enter the world in a hospital setting, making a hospital a location symbolically suited for becoming a parent. When a child is diagnosed with diabetes, the hospital takes on an instructional role, requiring the parent to actively practice new skills. The learner becomes a parent anew and redefines the world of family. Emerging from the hospitalization, the family has reconstructed a different kind of normal life through the pathway experience of hospitalization.

Reframed Notions of "Normal"

I'm so sick of the kids at school asking me questions. I want to get on the loudspeaker just one time, and yell to everybody, one time, and then have it done. 'Listen!' I'd yell. 'This is why I have to have a

snack, and test my blood, and get a shot, and everything. It's because of my diabetes. Stop asking me why, okay? It's because of my
diabetes. *Just stop asking me about it so much.'* That's what I'd say.
*I just want her to have an ordinary life like everybody else. I don't
think of her as sick at all. I want her to have a normal life. She can
do everything other kids do, except maybe become an airplane pilot as an adult. She can be a normal kid.*

Even children in perfect health rely on their parents to care
for them. Children with diabetes live in a world that is especially
closely monitored, persistently organized, and full of pricks and
pokes. In order for parents to exercise their responsibility toward
their diabetic child, a routine is scheduled and accommodated,
while full-fledged freedom gets set aside. Yet importantly, for the
accepting family, this constitutes a newly shared notion of "normal," in terms of parents' and child's ordinary expected reality.
Mothers stated that this post-diabetes life had now become the
norm. "That's our life now," one explained. Even one mother who
admitted to having the temperament of a "free spirit" by and large
had redefined life to normalize the rigors of diabetes management.
Mothers viewed their child's disease through a lens that excluded
stigmatizing, as far as they were concerned, since they viewed the
situation as normal. The arduous burdens of diabetes came to
be treated as matter-of-fact, as an automatic given in the child's
world, or as one child put it, "just regular." (When schoolmates
treated the routine as an odd curiosity by asking probing questions, this interrupted and on some level punctured the child's
matter-of-fact normality.)

Situation normal, as perceived by a child with diabetes, is
nevertheless a highly particular version of "normal." From the
diabetic child's perspective, the parent is never far from contact,
since it always seems to be time for some kind of intervention.
Among mothers who worked outside the home, telephones and

beepers provided ready accessibility. Maternal jobs were apt to be close to home or flexible enough to allow interruptions. When children started school, it was not unusual for a mother to visit school regularly, to administer a child's scheduled blood test or to volunteer—a guise for keeping tabs on the child. At home, mothers (and largely fathers, too) were ever mindful of their little one. Parents were ever aware of the clock and the scheduled times for food or insulin, monitoring the child's behavior for evidence of lows, assessing the impact of exercise on insulin and food needs when the weather was good enough for active play outside. As a matter of course, parents woke up in the wee hours to do an extra blood check when need be, so as to stave off an insulin reaction. Told of an upcoming celebration at school such as a birthday or holiday party, the parent stood ready to handle the situation so that their child would not be faced with a room full of forbidden treats; the mother might ask for or send in a substitute, permissible food. Parents seldom went out for social amusement, since it was hard to find reliable sitters or willing relatives who could or would handle the child's diabetes.

While these demands were heavy for the parent, for the child this behavior provided assurance of parental devotion. Children with diabetes could trust their parents' affection and reliability without question, since the parents' behavior gave ready, ubiquitous evidence.[16] Treatment may interrupt play, but it also signals maternal or parental affection, as children themselves articulated.

Looking at a photograph of himself doing his blood test with parental help, a six-year-old boy said, "That's another way of loving." A seven-year-old girl said the good part about diabetes is that "my mother has to help me. [That] makes me feel good, [like when] she helps me, um, does my blood test."

The close bond between diabetic children and their parents means that the adult caretaker is all the more equated with trust and safety during a child's earliest years. Children with diabetes said they view home as a "safe zone," and the parent as a sure, safe ally.[17] A mother, and many fathers, could be trusted to handle anything, including anxious moments, such as anxiety about being low. Children willingly cooperated with the demanding diabetes regimen largely as an adjunct of their trust in and affiliation with the ministering parent.

Parents did not believe that children used their diabetes as a direct bid for attention. Siblings of diabetic children likewise negated the notion that a chronically ill child would trade on the illness to gain attention. Rather than serving as an attention getter, diabetes provided affection as a by-product, in the course of shared family treatment activities. That is, parental devotion was implicitly perceived and appreciated by the child amidst treatment, as if parental love was emotionally sealed within the act of functional care. Parents dispensed hugs or kisses ("kissed it and made it better") along with requisite shots and blood tests, which helped soothe the child. This affection amidst treatment—tender loving care—was repeated through the child's lifeworld like clockwork, since occasions for treatment were so pervasive, and had come to be taken for granted as an ever-ready source of trust and security. In a sense, the parent-child bond was reinforced as steady and trustworthy due to the omnipresent procedures. For these young children, these procedures interrupted their play, but they also offered reassurance of parental reliability.

If diabetes carries any measure of content to family life, the benefit lies in the everyday heroism by which the regimen—treated within the family as ordinary—seals the bonds of family interconnection. As psychologist Kenneth Gorfinkle has written, a hurtful situation can become more tolerable and less upsetting to the whole family when the adult takes charge, exerts control, and conveys a sense of affectionate warmth.[18] Informants involved with diabetes would agree. Parental presence was said (by both parent and child) to make a child feel more secure at the doctor's

office, or hospital, or when getting an X-ray. When trusted familial affection (as opposed to clinical distancing) accompanied a
biomedical procedure or experience, the child's anxiety discernibly abated.[19]

Limits to Normality

When I started to do my own blood test, I was really proud. The
other kids thought I must be pretty brave to do that. Once I squirted
my blood at the bully down the street, during my blood test. He
ran away, fast, so I must be braver than him. Even my grandma
doesn't like to watch me do my blood test. I think it grosses her out.
But I'm proud I can do it. The part I don't like is not eating candy
and sugar. My mom made me a birthday cake I could eat, with
sugar-free Jell-O, so that was really good.

*I can bake a sugar-free birthday cake. But as far as I'm concerned,
Halloween is the dreaded holiday above all others. I could buy
sugarless candy for Easter. And at Christmas the kids get toys, not
candy. But at Halloween, he wants to go trick-or-treating. He comes
home and trades his candy for money. I got that idea, to buy his
Halloween candy, at a meeting of my mothers' support group, at
the clinic. Our support group is always talking about ideas for parties and holidays, and how to get around problems.*

The notion that a child with diabetes can live a fully "normal" life in all social domains—optimistically voiced by mothers
and medical caretakers—runs up against experience in children's
everyday social affairs. Children with diabetes cannot eat as flexibly as other children, due to the need to eat a planned diet on a
planned schedule. When they start school, for example, their rigid
eating schedule directly contrasts with that of other children, ex-
posing the ruse of assumed normality when curious peers query
the child about why he eats a snack when no one else does. The

rhythm of the diabetic child's daily life is uncharacteristically rigid, especially in a culture permeated by on-the-run, spur-of-the-moment fast food. Moreover, even within the permitted rhythm, dietary choices are restricted. At times, young informants admitted to using the system itself to break the pattern, pretending to feel low to get an extra sweet. Mothers were apt to catch on quickly to such shenanigans, though, subsequently giving a blood test before acting on a child's claim to be low. When school events or parties involving food were planned, a mother would typically send along a permissible snack as a substitute. Yet this parental effort to normalize the social event failed to completely compensate; forbidden treats, in excessive quantities, still taunted and tempted amid the festive setting of a social gathering. In private, several youngsters admitted to me they had sneaked candy at a picnic, or ice cream at a festival, or treats at some other social event. Mothers also told of telltale signs of pilfered treats, such as red-colored tongues or unexpected highs on blood tests.

At times of festivity, social sharing can call for indulgence, which makes preserving normality a dilemma for both diabetic child and mother. Some mothers tried to work desired treats into the diet as part of the overall plan, including a chance for one girl to taste a marshmallow while camping with friends. Another mother recorded her dilemma in her field notes, regarding a party: "Today was the graduation party. It is so hard to limit Tom's snacking when there is a party. . . . It is just so hard to say no all the time. I just figure Tom's readings will be a little high today and he will enjoy himself." This same mother's seven-year-old son was saddened by the mere illustration of a birthday cake during an interview: "I feel sad [when I see the picture of cake] 'cause I usually won't get the frosting, and a lot of people would." Festive occasions gain their expressive meaning, through the symbolism of food, among other things. By eating, the participant literally internalizes shared social meaning.[20] Sweet foods, such as a wedding cake or

Valentine's Day chocolates, can carry meanings of affection. Abundant amounts of food carry social significance, as when Thanksgiving dinner guests stuff themselves (with stuffing and also other goodies) as a celebration of material plenty.[21] School pizza parties or birthday cakes are opportunities for shared exuberance through eating.

Bearing in mind the symbolic, expressive role of food, it follows that even though a child may be nurtured physically through a controlled diet, the young eater nevertheless can feel out of balance socially or expressively. Food signifies social relatedness.[22] From an outing to the baseball park with its ritual song lyrics, "Buy me some peanuts and Cracker Jacks," or the jingling arrival of an ice cream truck in the neighborhood, to participating in a school bake sale, decorating holiday cookies, or enjoying cotton candy at the circus, diabetic children are disadvantaged in their full, expressive participation and belonging. The pain of this food-derived stigma is palpable.

An eight-year-old boy commented, looking at a picture of an airplane: "You're, like, flying, and the waitress gives you something to eat. If there's candy you can't have it. That's, like, the most biggest sad part on the plane." A six-year-old boy said: "At my brother's baseball games, they give out treats. . . . At my brother's All Star game my sister got some cookies and I didn't." And the mother of a six-year-old son reported that her son said: " 'I'm not going to go [trick or treating] this year because I never eat all the candy anyway, so why go. I don't want to go.' And he didn't go and he just handed out candy."

When children imagined a cure for diabetes—a pervasive fantasy appropriated by many children and families—their idealizations were the proverbial "visions of sugar plums." Only in fantasy could children participate fully in the eating of festive, indulgent food, restraint thrown aside. Wishing for a cure was not rare. Presented with a wish-invoking opportunity—blowing out birthday candles, throwing a coin into a fountain, writing a letter to Santa, or breaking the wishbone from a poultry dinner—the choice of appropriate wish was obvious to diabetic children.

> BOY (age eight): I would be happy if they had a cure for diabetes.
> CDC: You would? What would you do the day after you got your cure?
> BOY: My mama would let me have all the candy I wanted. . . .
> I could have regular pop, all kinds. Usually I drink this drink.
> [Points to can of diet cola] [If] the diabetic eats candy, he can die, like.

Some diabetic youngsters enjoyed playing the game Candyland, a manufactured board game in which one travels through a candy-filled world. Ironically, a group of children played the Candyland game during the meetings of a local diabetic parents support group. At home, kindergartner Jenny brought out Candyland during our interview and asked me to join her in playing it, much to her enjoyment. Through fantasy play about candy, diabetic children reverse (and reveal) their starvation for indulgence, their sense of expressive undernourishment. That is, they play at or imagine the indulgent eating they miss. Using their capacity to fantasize a better alternative to the diabetic routine, children improvise their own play therapy (a form of "imaginal coping," a topic of Chapter 4).

Halloween, as a festival, particularly accentuates the social and expressive price of the diabetic diet. Children grumbled in interviews about being diabetic at Halloween, despite receiving money from parents in trade for their trick-or-treat candy. Parents, feeling that money was an adequate substitute for treats, were typically shielded from (and unaware of) the extent of their children's Halloween angst. In private with me, children complained bitterly.

Halloween hit especially hard in the Brent family, in which

two brothers were both diabetic. Richard Brent had been diagnosed at age thirteen months and was eight years old at the time of the study. His brother, Roger, was ten years old and had been diagnosed at age five. My second visit to the boys' urban home occurred shortly after Halloween. Since July, the family had been keeping a research record about daily life with diabetes, at my request. The events at Halloween were recorded in Mrs. Brent's field notes, and also in photographs taken by the boys. Mrs. Brent's field notes, recorded on Halloween day, reported that the day had not been completely enjoyable for the Brent brothers.

> Halloween—The parties at school were difficult for both children. There was so much candy, cake and fruit, it looked like a sweet table at a wedding.
>
> Once again I let the boys go trick-or-treating, and said I would *buy* their bags of candy. They opted to keep it—we soon started arguing as to whether I would give them any money at all.
>
> It is very difficult for them and I become very angry since they cannot eat the candy like other children.
>
> At the end of the day, they were tired and wanted to eat the candy. They started to cry and say they did *not* want to have diabetes.

The family had taken photographs of an abundant array of sweets available at the school Halloween party, arranged buffet style. At the buffet, children took their plates and walked along to add what they wanted (or, in the case of the diabetic child, what he was allowed) to their plates. The buffet was brimfull of sweet treats forbidden on Richard's diet, and Richard moved along with a nearly empty plate. Other photos displayed the bittersweet process of sorting the plunder Richard gained from trick-or-treating; the boys handled the candy piece by piece, picking out the nonsugar candy or pretzels or other foods permitted within their strictly controlled diet. As he sorted, Roger confessed to feeling "bad" because "when you smell it, it makes you want to eat it." His brother agreed, saying, "You want to stick your face in it and eat it." Throughout trick-or-treating, they complained, they thought about the candy they couldn't eat, rather than the money for which they would trade the candy to their parents. "You're crying 'cause you see all the candy and you want it so bad," one brother admitted. They agreed that they would prefer to "push away" the sweets altogether. These brothers normally wore a school uniform to school and were happy that they got to "dress up" on Halloween day, and to have some money at the end of it all. But their complaints about forbidden candy predominated in their discussion of Halloween, ceasing only when their mother wisely intervened in our interview to change the subject to a potential cure for diabetes.

In some ways, the Brent brothers, like other diabetic children, masqueraded twice on Halloween. Their visible masquerade was the costume, such as Richard's football player outfit. Their unseen masquerade was that, in effect, they were "passing" as trick-or-treaters rather than fully playing the role.[23] Children, usually powerless relative to adults, ritually threaten to "trick" adults at Halloween unless appeased with treats.[24] This ritualized role reversal holds particular attraction for diabetic children. The assertion of power at Halloween—the inverted act of children laying claim to adult-controlled candy—is especially attractive for the child with diabetes, who is daily dominated by adult dictates authorized by medical fiat. Yet for the diabetic child, the role reversal is effectively rendered impotent at the close of Halloween night. The directive to relinquish collected treats to parental control, albeit in exchange for money, reasserts adult power over childish indulgence. The promise of Halloween turns out to be as hollow as cheap candy, one more form of indulgence denied the child with diabetes.

Depending upon the sensitive adjustments of adults, a diabetic youngster's Halloween experience can be ameliorated. A seven-year-old girl, Alice, provides an example of how diabetic children can be singled out by for differential treatment on Halloween by thoughtful adults who modify sweet treats. Field notes kept by Alice's mother illustrate:

HALLOWEEN

The hardest holiday of the year. I sent a bag to school for her treat bag filled with different kinds of stickers, tattoos, necklaces, etc.—all non-edible. And when she came home—she, without a second thought, handed over any candy she received to Daddy and me. She displayed her treasures and her sister and brother *never* showed an ounce of *jealousy.* Alice was so excited—her room mom made a special sugar free "pudding grave yard" just like the other kids' grave yard snack. [The school nurse] gave her a special Halloween mug, and the assistant principal gave her a sugar free muffin.

Well Dad took the kids out [trick or treating] in the rain before and after dinner. . . . Most neighbors had things just for Alice—i.e. sugar free Fannie May's [brand candy], sugar free gum, and one neighbor even made her a balloon [arrangement]. . . . She brought home two big bags of candy—and turned it all over to us. I guess this is a ritual—none of the kids get to "keep" their candy, and *everyone* must ask for permission to have a piece.

Alice benefited from an unusually considerate network of adults who took trouble to provide her with sugarless treats permissible in her diet. Yet Alice's sugared treats nevertheless were inspected and selectively confiscated by her parents. The lack of jealousy by her siblings over her special sugarless treats hints that Alice's "special" treatment did not in the final analysis carry coveted status. Alice had no control over the non-option of eating sweets.

Mothers shared a consensus, perhaps a somewhat self-misleading one. They believed their diabetic children enjoyed trick-or-treating, despite the trade-in required at night's close. The maternal version of events overlooked the social, expressive sustenance encoded in sugary Halloween treats—the notion of candies as symbolic expressions of juvenile power. Mothers did not always realize that, as seen through young diabetic eyes, the ultimate payoff of the bounty of Halloween is bittersweet at best; the role reversal of Halloween by which youth demand treats from adults is cut short by the adult parents' control and confiscation of the sweet rewards. Halloween's rituals promise more than gets delivered to the diabetic child. These children learn that diabetes carries a social penalty, that they are singled out to be different, that they cannot escape being non-normative, that they cannot "pass" as normal through all situations. Festival, normally a means of group sharing and cohesion, sets the diabetic child apart as stigmatized, even while the child attempts to participate.

Grider has pointed out that Halloween may be one of the first holidays in which a school-age child participates with nonfamily members.[25] The symbolism of Halloween (skeletons, witches, and other things that frighten) provides a platform for practicing bravery, a skill at which the diabetic child excels, being well accustomed to the sight of blood and the sensation of pain—not to mention the intersection of life and death. But instead of reinforcing a sense of exceptional heroism, Halloween ultimately reminds the diabetic child of the deprivation and stigma of being exceptional.

Stigma is not in fact a fixed component of having an illness but rather a byproduct of interacting social dynamics, we learn from the case study of the diabetic trick-or-treater. It is because the child is unable to engage socially in normative ways that the child is stigmatized. Stigma is an actively charged state brought about through social activity, not a reducible, fixed component of the child's personality. This distinction is profound, for it requires us to think about suffering and coping in more dynamic, interpersonal terms. To address the stress caused by diabetes, one must reassess the dynamics of birthday parties, Halloween, school social interplay, outings of all kinds, and interactions with neighbors, friends, and relations. Stigma is to be found in customary and improvised activity, energized by social interaction.

Blood, Shots, and Tears

Yesterday, my grandmother was staying with us. It's funny, whenever I do my insulin shot around her, she walks out of the room. I think she gets grossed out. She came to watch my soccer game at night, and I had to do my shot at the soccer field. It's funny, the coach walked away when I did my shot, too. But my friends stay around during my shot, when they're here. Once I took a picture of my shot, see? This friend looked like she was flinching when the needle went in. I never noticed her doing that around me, until now.

I don't know what he says, but I think he's gotten used to the shots by now. Most of the time it's no big deal to him. He only complains sometimes. It's been a couple of years. He must be used to it.

Whether or not parents were aware of it, children with diabetes harbored dislike toward injections, although the dislike was not necessarily proclaimed to all. In private interviews, children said that shots engendered a combination of dread, anger, hurt, or fear. "Having to take injections" was a pronounced dislike, a finding consistent with an earlier investigation that uncovered an even greater dislike for shots than for dietary restrictions.[26] Shots cause pain, not only on a physical level but also on an emotional, expressive level. However sterile and efficiently delivered, injections do violence to the boundaries of self.

Requested to do so during interviews, children sorted through pictures of objects, such as a bee, a teddy bear, a witch, a life jacket, a treasure chest, a rod of lightning, and an airplane. Children chose objects they thought had a similar mood or feeling to each treatment, blood test, or injection. Based on evidence from this Metaphor Sort Test (MST), an insulin injection had negative associations and meanings to children. A "shot" was repeatedly compared to such disliked entities as the "sting" of a bee, the "bite" of a spider, the "scary" feeling of lightning, the "boom" of a bomb, or a "mean," "bad" witch who harms. Even though feelings of safety—"keeping you alive"— were associated with insulin by a minority, these positive feelings were apt to coexist with misgivings. An injection of insulin comprises a painful intrusion that invades the child in an intimate, unwelcome way.

By comparison, a blood-glucose check presents a less hurtful procedure than an injection, as children described. While the idea of a blood test might have seemed scary at the beginning (with the loss of blood, in principle, a cause for fear), with experience, children by their own report became acclimated to blood testing. Indeed, blood tests were repeatedly compared in the MST sorting to protective, safe objects, such as a "snuggly" teddy bear, or the "safe" protection of an umbrella or bicycle helmet. To show how a blood test gave a "safe" feeling like an umbrella, one boy held the picture of the umbrella over his head, explaining that the blood test kept him protected like the umbrella and made it easier to balance, just as an umbrella did when walking a "tightrope." A blood test brought reassurance to children, a way to stay in safe balance, whereas insulin was less credited with reassurance. A blood test did not sting and pierce in the painful way of injected insulin. Undoubtedly it is also relevant that several children did their own blood tests, controlling this act at an early age prior to learning to self-inject insulin.

Faced with a ceaseless routine of blood tests and disliked shots, children told me they had developed personal rituals, idiosyncratic actions that habitually accompanied a treatment. Such rituals were especially common in the case of injections. Through

personal rituals, children found a way to direct or control the necessarily painful experience of being injected. For example, one
five-year-old girl liked to cover her mother's ears during a shot—
perhaps signifying a cry not made and unheard. Some diabetic
siblings liked getting shots together. A girl with a diabetic cat liked
to get her shot alongside her pet, which received insulin using the
same syringe, after the girl's shot was finished. Some children adjusted their breathing while injecting, with two variations: breathing slowly and steadily or, alternatively, holding the breath until
the shot was over. Special ways of pushing in the needle were used
by some diabetic children, such as, in one case, using a special automatic injecting device that pushed the needle in when a button
was pushed. In another instance, the ministering parent allowed
the child to complete the last step, to push in the syringe manually.
When a child learned to self-inject entirely, the child's claimed discomfort lessened with achievement of full personal control.

Rituals also took place after the injection. A few children
wore a reassuring plastic bandage over the site, chosen from
among store-purchased character-decorated designs. One boy, as
a toddler, hit his mother after each shot. Others after each injection preferred a rub, a hug, a scream or shout, or being rocked.

Rituals have been said to provide "frameworks for expec-
tancy" through the familiarity of repetition and predictability,
such as covering the mother's ear, during every shot.[27] Rituals allow strong emotions to be contained or safely expressed without
leading to social disharmony.[28] Mother-child relations might be
disrupted by a child's cry during an injection, for example, but not
if the child covers the mother's ears instead of crying.

One mother and five-year-old son shared in pretend play
during each insulin treatment by jointly imagining that the syringe with its demarcated lines of measurement was a zebra. The
mother pretended that the zebra "kissed" the boy (when injecting),

expressively preserving the notion that this intrusion was an act of love. The child was invited to hit or dismantle (i.e., destroy) the "bad" syringe-zebra afterwards, as an outlet for negative feelings about such a hurtful "kiss." In effect, the zebra game allowed mother-child harmony to remain intact, while encoding the emotional misgivings of both parties.

In undergoing a medical procedure, children are in effect asked to surrender their body to invasive adult control, often with no account taken of the child's preferences in the matter.[29] The child's need to retain or regain some form of control reveals itself through personal ritualized behaviors. Physicians encourage rotation of sites to avoid uneven absorption due to tissue build up.[30] Yet diabetic children are widely known to develop a preference for a particular injection site, another means of keeping dominion over their own body.[31] Based on my research, children resist relinquishing jurisdiction about where a shot is given. "Ted will not do his insulin anymore in the thigh. Now the only places are the stomach and hip," wrote the mother of a six-year-old in her field notes.

A father of six- and eleven-year-old brothers said: "Mike likes his in his arms, and Ed doesn't like it in his arms. Ed likes it in his belly. Obviously you gotta change, off and on, but I give Ed either in his belly or his leg, and Mike, . . . all his shots in his arms."

The mother of a five-year-old reported: "He says, 'I don't want it in the tummy.' [I say that] 'we're going to discuss this with your doctor. You can talk to the doctor about where you want your shots.'"

However well intentioned, adults ask much when, during hurtful intrusions, they subvert children's sense of control over their bodies. The child views this issue symbolically and expressively rather than biomedically. For the body is symbolically equated with self. The body mediates the nature of a child's self and relationships. The unseen malfunctioning of internal tissue is less important and less understood by the child than the visible body's surface integrity and self-identity. Injections violate and disrupt the intact bodily self, issuing a call for the child to somehow regain self-integrity and control. The resistance to site rotation serves the child's desire for some degree of control over his person, as when one child declared, "I like to do my stomach in the morning and my hip at night."

Writing about the soothing of pain, psychologist Gorfinkle stated the case for a sensitive understanding of injections:

> It is very easy for us adults to minimize or deny the non-physical (emotional and cognitive) contributors to a child's pain. If we feel guilty for putting the child through the ordeal, we fall into the pattern of belief that the only real pain is from the mechanical effect of the needle puncturing the skin. We want to say "Now that wasn't so bad, was it?" or, "How brave you were!" in our efforts to convey the wish to remove the child's fear and anxiety from the equation and diminish the pain. And sure enough children hear our wishes and learn to suppress their feelings next time.[32]

In the families of children with diabetes, parents cooperated, where possible, with desired rituals. In so doing they were, to a significant extent, accommodating the child's feelings and need to have control over fears. West African scholar and healer Malidoma Somé has written that ritual is the "anti-machine" in the modern world, since ritual by nature has a different rhythm than mechanized entities and addresses needs which the machines of "progress" neglect. Somé asserts that the creative process of ritual can ensure wholeness amidst the tyranny of modern mechanization.[33] Children, pressing for the predictable, playful rhythms of ritual amidst treatment by syringe, push against passivity and toward human control and intactness. Parental support in this encounter recognizes that human needs, and not just mechanics, are valued.

Anthropologists Sjaak Van der Geest and Susan Whyte have argued that medications do symbolic work because they are concrete substances; medications render an illness graspable, treatable, and formative of particular social relations (given the social arrangements by which medication is dispensed).[34] Treatment devices have social and expressive dimensions, as well as technological dimensions.[35] For instance, as discussed earlier, children view concrete forms of treatment such as injections and blood tests almost as defining diabetes. Testing blood-glucose levels and injecting insulin are socially meaningful, since these activities engender and signal a close social bond between parent-injector and child. Yet, treatments invade life and body when fun activity must yield to relentlessly recurrent "poking."

Ultimately, treatments serve as social, expressive opportunities through which the child's needs can be either recognized or ignored. While children have no control over having diabetes, they can and do seek some control over the concrete, felt impact of treatment. They cannot, as Mary Poppins suggested, have a spoonful of sugar to make the medicine go down; for them, this is not a dietary option. But they can amuse themselves in other ways, such as through a "wager" (with a diabetic uncle) about what the blood-glucose test number will be, a "race" (with a diabetic sibling) to see who can draw and test blood fastest, or a make-believe narrative that the blood testing machine is actually a blood-sucking polar bear, to name a few examples. Juvenile attempts to insert a Poppins-like element of enjoyment into treatment are one way children stay "brave" and in control amidst the physiological and social pain. Playful and ritual practices help to favorably reframe the treatments' intrusions within the creative and expressive milieu of child-mediated activity. In other words, children insert symbolic, expressive meaning into treatment, as will be discussed in more detail in Chapter 4.

Feeling Low

No way, no. I don't want to stop roller-blading now. I don't want to.

I'm grabbing you because you seem low. I have glucose tablets right here in my pocket. Open your mouth and sit still.

Hypoglycemia (known in the diabetic vernacular as a "low") is a well-known medical emergency affecting children with diabetes.[36] Sometimes called an insulin reaction, since it can occur from receiving too much insulin, a low can be caused by an unexpected boost in exercise, by not having eaten enough food, and by an infection or (according to mothers) rapid growth. A low can occur without much warning. Signs that a child is low include unusual changes in behavior or mood (such as irritability or lost concentration), or a subjective feeling of "strangeness" by the child. Nightmares can accompany nocturnal low reactions. Dizziness, shakiness, headaches, and poor coordination are among the other symptoms, each potentially upsetting to children. The same child may feel slightly different each time she is low. The experience carries a woozy unsteadiness that can make children (or for that matter, adults) ill at ease.[37]

An insulin reaction introduces the uncontrollable into a child's world: unpredictable symptoms, altered thinking, and sensations conveying a rupture of steady-state stability. The subjective feeling was compared by one girl to the experience of riding a roller coaster, which she drew for me on paper to illustrate the wavering unevenness, the woozy pattern of ups and downs. Another child likened being low to being on a boat, swaying with the choppy water. When children wake up low during the night, they can be frightened, themselves, and frightening to parents. The effort of parents to reverse a nighttime reaction might well be accompanied by a cranky, upset, and uncooperative child, unable to make sense of the situation.

One mother described a nighttime low in her field notes:

THURSDAY MIDNIGHT—
I woke up to David crying and having a bad reaction. By the time I got to him, he was unable to drink juice. I woke up my husband and we both started to help David out of his reaction. He could not drink juice. He started biting the straw. I tried to gently squeeze the juice into his mouth but he just would bite the straw. I ran to get a sugar packet, placing some sugar on the inside of his lip. He bit my finger, so we tried to give him juice. After one hour, he was starting to feel better. He knew who we were, but did not realize he had a reaction. Needless to say, we were *all* very exhausted. And the day after, he spent on the couch or in the bathroom vomiting. He was worn out from the night before.

A mother of a seven-year-old boy described a nighttime low away from home:

The one time was at our church camp. . . . We were gonna get up at six and leave [for home], but at four o'clock I heard him, and he was making funny sounds up in his bed. Everything was packed. . . . I [said] "Well, Mike, you gotta go to the bathroom?" He just let out a gurgle sound—a grunt almost. It was not a word. And then I got scared. He's never been to . . . that point before. . . . This time he got beyond shaky. I called my husband, he happened to be there that night. . . . [I said to my husband] "You gotta get here right now." Cause the kid was on the top bunk. Three bunks up. "You just gotta get him down!"

The mother laughed, in hindsight, at the predicament of a low child in a high bunk bed.

So we got him down. And I gave him some juice without even taking his [blood-sugar] number. And then I took his number and it was still really low. He went back to sleep and then he started throwing up . . . so you're in this Catch-22 circle. . . . [Sometimes] he'll get up in the morning, and I think he's fine. But all the sudden he—he's not. He'll come up and try to talk to us and he's not making sense. And my husband and I are looking at each other, and your heart starts pounding.

If trauma is "a sudden, extraordinary, external event" that "overwhelms an individual's capacity to cope and master the feelings aroused," an insulin reaction can be a kind of recurring trauma (albeit a reversible one) in the lifeworld of diabetes.[38] At root, human attention and thought control diabetes through the monitoring of blood sugar and the dosing and timing of insulin, food, and exercise. An insulin reaction may interfere with the diabetic's thinking and attention, rendering a situation out of balance without warning. Even though claiming a low can allow a child to indulge in some form of sugar (as a medicinal measure), a full-fledged severe reaction with changed consciousness and physical symptoms can make a child uneasy or frightened. A low child, not to mention the ministering parents, is thrown out of kilter. A low child might be offered a usually desirable sugared soda and yet irrationally refuse to drink it. A low crisis exposes as less than total the illusion of balance carefully tuned day-to-day through treatment. The sight of a child shivering, crying, and perhaps unable to talk reminds everyone in the family, siblings and ill child included, of the potential for danger. Lows can be treated, but they nevertheless leave behind traces of a basic unsteadiness, for child and family alike.

Identity Bracelets

I never want to take off my bracelet that says I have diabetes.

*The doctor says you should always wear it. When you get too big
for it, we'll get a bigger one so you can always wear it.*

Along with following the prescribed diet and treatment regimen, diabetics are encouraged to wear a medical identification
tag. The medical alert tag, worn in the form of an ID bracelet or
necklace, is meant to inform others of the need for lifesaving treatment in an emergency. Identification jewelry worn every day by
children holds expressive meaning apart from its precautionary
purpose. First of all, ID jewelry is literally a signal of being diabetic.
If a person is without such jewelry, it follows that the individual
does not have diabetes. "She don't have diabetes or she would be
wearing this thing," one boy reasoned about his endocrinologist,
pointing to his own ID necklace. For their own part, youngsters
generally did not resent being tagged as diabetic. On the contrary,
the identification jewelry was to many young wearers a source of
serenity and even an inherent facet of identity.

"She wears that [bracelet] at all times," said the mother of a
seven-year-old. "That never comes off. . . . It's her. . . . It's part of
her. . . . She doesn't play with it. You know, I play with my watch.
I don't see her playing with it. She was asked at the beginning of
soccer to remove it, cause they don't want jewelry. And she said
'No, I don't take this off.' And they came to me and I said 'No.' We
held the meeting to make sure everybody realized that if a child or
somebody is wearing it, you don't ask them to remove it."

Among preschoolers who attended a day camp for diabetes,
their shared status as diabetic was vividly apparent through identification jewelry. The researcher/counselor's field notes for August 7, 1995, report: "As the kids were waiting to have their blood
sugars drawn on the first day of camp, they started comparing jewelry. One of the older counselors, Louis, had a necklace. Keith
asked Louis about the necklace—why he had it instead of a brace-

let. Alice, who was very proud of her bracelet, wanted to show it to me. She had gotten it a month before for her sixth birthday."

The security symbolized by ID jewelry was evident in the feelings of safety children professed about it. "You never have to take it off, so you feel better," was how one boy expressed it. At times, the standard ID bracelet was further decorated, when the child put something else on the same chain. John had a crucifix hanging chained to his ID tag, ensuring him that "God is with me." Being able to "count on" God (emblematically part of his emergency jewelry) and to know that "if I get in a crash, people will know I have diabetes" gave John double reassurance. Another boy, Ted, had an ID tag shaped like military dog tags, which had been special-ordered by his mother. Wearing a pendant similar to dog tags popular in cosmetic jewelry, Ted felt "cool" and even "gutsy."

Perhaps, the ready acceptance of ID jewelry gives evidence that at these young ages, children accepted their diabetes, by and large, as part of their identity. Most of the young children in this study knew other children with diabetes, through school, family, support group, or camp—thereby realizing that diabetes was a shared fate. The stress of diabetes was attached more to its treatment regimen than to being labeled diabetic. Being singled out and stigmatized could be traced to social experiences—lack of conformity with festive eating practices, interruptions of play for blood checks and shots, and so on—rather than to strict self-labeling. As already discussed, interrupted play, intrusive "pokes" and shots, and the inability to share festive, indulgent eating of treats all carried a sense of disruption or deprivation. Stigma is not intrinsically attached to being diabetic, then, as much as it comes from the isolating, exceptionalizing processes that accompany treatment.

In the final analysis, the readiness with which diabetic children wore jewelry labeling themselves as such (and their security when so adorned) is an observable testament to these families' adjustment to a new kind of normal life, that is, "diabetic but still normal." Aided by the rite of passage of hospitalization and empowered by their competence at treatment, diabetic families bring a tour de force of family resolve against the daily challenge of diabetes. As will be seen in Chapter 3, such thorough acceptance and adjustment are not equally typical of all chronic illness.

Enduring Childhood Asthma

Invisible though it is, air is a very real substance. . . . So
necessary is air to the maintenance of life that it has not
been left to us to control our use of it as we do in the case of
food and drink. Unconsciously, and with no volition on our
part, we admit the air to our lungs and allow it to play its
wonderful part in our system. On air, more than anything
else, we live, our daily bread taking only second place. Our
need of food is felt only at comparatively long intervals; the
need of air is felt uninterruptedly, ever imperious, even
inexorable.   JOHN HENRI FABRE

What is the length of a human life?
One inhalation and one exhalation.

SHAKAYAMUNI BUDDHA

If you don't breathe you can die.

SIX-YEAR-OLD BOY WITH ASTHMA

*A*sthma has become almost a commonplace illness, affecting
far more children than does diabetes. Based on 2001 estimates,
only 1.2 children per thousand had diabetes, while fifty-three children out of a thousand had asthma.[1] Furthermore, the prevalence
of childhood asthma is increasing.[2] Asthma is the most common
reason for children being admitted to pediatric hospitals; the rate
of hospitalization has risen dramatically over recent decades.[3]
Asthma causes more school absences than any other illness.[4] Although physicians view asthma as a manageable, reversible illness,
the death rate from asthma has been on the rise.[5] In 1996, 293
deaths of U.S. children under nineteen were attributed to asthma.[6]

Asthma: Some Background

Breathing, while essential to life, is a process most of us take for granted. Passages known as airways automatically carry air to the air sacs of our lungs, where blood is oxygenated—all without our giving the process a second thought. For a non-asthmatic person, breathing is a life-giving process challenged only under acute circumstances. If exposed to excessive smoke from a fire, for example, even a healthy person will cough and splutter; irritation in the lining of the airways, along with the formation of mucus, elicits coughing to clear the airway passages.

In a person with asthma, the airways are hyperreactive, so they become inflamed in response to seemingly modest irritants. In allergic asthma, substances that would normally not affect breathing (dust mites, pet hair, pollens, etc.) can produce an extensive hyperreactive response. The linings of the airways swell, excessive amounts of mucus are produced, and the smooth-muscle tissue of the airways tightens or constricts.

Due to asthma, then, the airways through which air travels to the air sacs narrow in response to triggering substances. They become swollen and irritated, and further irritants (such as environmental tobacco smoke, air pollution, or chemical fumes) are all the more apt to breed additional reactivity, swelling, and mucus. One feature of the asthmatic response is its cumulative, accruing impact; once the airways are reactive, the threshold for additional problems is all the more sensitive. Asthmatic response paves the way for more asthmatic response, in a vicious cycle of inflammation and breathlessness.

Numerous factors can trigger an asthmatic reaction, as Nancy Sander has summarized.[7] The founder of a national support organization for parents of children with asthma, Sander lists the following activators or irritants. Bear in mind that a given child with asthma may not respond to every activator, and that this list may leave out triggers that affect certain individuals.

- colds and infections
- exercise
- mold
- tree or grass pollen
- certain foods and additives
- animals (especially dogs, cats, birds, horses)
- wind, rain, cold air
- dramatic fluctuations in weather
- aspirin
- beta-blockers
- aerosol sprays
- odors
- smoke
- dust
- air pollution
- paint fumes
- perfume
- laughing, crying
- holding breath
- hyperventilating

Asthmatic children and their families, as part of medical treatment, are encouraged to identify which activators bring on the child's attacks, and to make adjustments to avoid or minimize problems in the child's environment and activities.[8] For example, a child might use an inhaled medication before exercising, if she is subject to exercise-induced attacks. Or a youngster might avoid sleeping over at a friend's whose pet's hair triggers asthma. Still, not all activators can be avoided, since some are inherently uncontrollable. The most common cause of an attack of asthma is a viral infection, especially common in late fall and winter, with exposure unavoidable in the social context of school.[9]

Some environmental triggers require extensive changes in the home, such as removing draperies or carpeting to control dust. Parental smoking is another proven trigger for many young patients.[10] Children living with two parents who smoke have a 9 percent chance of having asthma, in contrast to a 4.5 percent chance if only one parent smokes and a 1.5 percent chance if no parent is a smoker. These statistics provide a strong inducement for an asthmatic child's parent to stop smoking.[11] Despite the patent risk, however, many parents of asthmatic children continue to smoke (including several parents of children in this study). In short, not all triggers are eliminated in all families.

The medical regimen prescribed for asthma is generally tailored to the needs of the particular child. The treatment plan takes into account what triggers the asthma and whether attacks are short term (with normal lung function in between) or whether there is continuous, prolonged wheezing. For the majority of children, asthma is a mild episodic problem. But a small proportion of children have chronic severe asthma. (The children followed in this research had chronic severe asthma, since study participants were screened on that basis.)[12]

Medications for childhood asthma come in several forms. The widely familiar "puffer," or metered-dose inhaler, used to treat adult asthma is not a universal form of treatment for young children. Metered-dose inhaling requires tots to regulate their inhalation simultaneously with dispensing a puff of medicine, which can be difficult for preschoolers to coordinate. Children younger than two generally receive their medication through means that allow them to breathe in and out at will, such as a nebulizer, a machine that uses tubing and a face mask and delivers the premeasured medication continuously. Older children and adults also use nebulizers. While inhaling through the nebulizer, a person must sit still for a prolonged period.

Additionally, children older than age two can use a spacer device; a metered-dose inhaler delivers the medicine to the spacer device, and the child inhales the medicine through a one-way valve in the spacer for five to ten seconds, rather than directly through the inhaler. This helps to ensure complete delivery of the medication. Among the children with severe asthma who participated in this study, many used a spacer especially designed for children, known by the brand name Inspirease. The Inspirease spacer is made of light-blue plastic, including a soft collapsible plastic compartment that fills up with air and then recedes, accordion-style, as the child inhales and exhales. This allows the child to inhale the medicine fully without the necessity to coordinate their breathing with the metered-dose device.

Another piece of equipment familiar to allergy or pulmonary specialists is the peak-flow meter, used to monitor the child's asthma and to catch early signs of deterioration or improvement. The child, typically five or older, exhales fully into the peak-flow meter, yielding a numerical measure of "peak flow" or maximum exhalation. If the child's peak flow drops precipitously, medications can be adjusted to give relief.

Medications for asthma are varied as well as complex. Some medicines are bronchodilators that open the airways to make breathing easier. Some medicines, such as corticosteroids, reduce inflammation. Some, such as cromolyn, interfere with the histamine release that is part of the allergic-reaction process. Some prescribed drugs work immediately and would be appropriate for reversing an attack; others work in a long-term or preventative fashion. The same medication may come as oral remedy (in liquid form, to be taken by mouth), for inhaling by metered-dose inhaler, or for the nebulizer.

A child with severe asthma may take several medications,

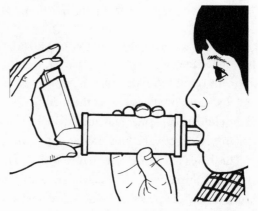

1. A child uses an inhaler with a spacer device

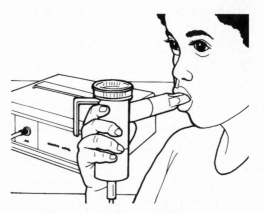

2. A child uses a machine nebulizer

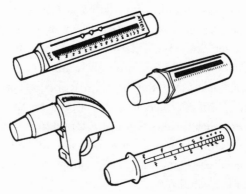

3. Versions of peak-flow measurement devices

each addressing a different aspect of the disease process. When I visited the homes of severely asthmatic children, families showed me large stores of medicines and supplies prescribed to be used according to the pattern of effectiveness. Full kitchen cabinets stocked with medicines, spacers, nebulizer, nebulizer face masks, and tubing were not ususual. Across the various medications, side effects can (and according to our informants, do) occur, with incidence and severity that differ from child to child. The medical management of severe asthma, in short, is complex, encompassing a variety of approaches and forms, potential side effects, and the simultaneous use of multiple remedies.

Asthma's Impact

I don't know what would be the cure for asthma. I just know if I got cured, I would sing a happy song and sing it loud and long. I'd be able to breathe better, so I could sing all I wanted. Because I wouldn't cough any more like I do all the time. And I wouldn't have to take so much medicine morning, day, and night.

Asthma is just one of the trials of life. There are a lot of hardships, but it could be worse, if she had a more serious illness like cancer. I figure she'll outgrow it, and that will be that. I don't think about curing asthma, really.[13]

Asthma is anything but clear-cut. As experienced by sufferers and families, persistent asthma has an indeterminate quality, even elusive and foglike, since irregularity and obscurity characterize the triggering factors, the pattern of symptoms, and the efficacy of treatments. No two asthmatic children respond precisely the same way to medications and activators. The same child may experience pronounced changes in the asthmatic response from one day to the next, one season to the next, and one year to the next. Compared to diabetes, asthma is a shifting, obscure entity:

harder to pin down, changing form from case to case, and caused by myriad stubbornly interlocking factors that are difficult to control all at once.

Despite available treatments, visits to the emergency room are commonplace, especially for an asthma episode that is out of control or worsening. In a Philadelphia survey, it was found that one-third of children with asthma had visited a hospital emergency room during the preceding year. In line with asthma's complex treatment, parents at the hospital were in many cases found to have administered a key medication incorrectly, or to have misunderstood the doctor's prescribed treatment plan. Such miscommunication can and does cause fatalities. In recent years, the number of Americans of all ages who die of asthma reaches into the thousands annually.[14]

Asthma has been called an "invisible and unpredictable chronic illness" that can frighten even adult patients as they helplessly struggle for air "like a fish out of water."[15] The phantom-like (since unseen and indeterminate) challenge to breathing, the symptoms that arise without appointment or predictability, and the nondefinitive, multifaceted treatment all make for a disease that can be frightening and elusive—and all the while as impalpable as air itself.

Even the diagnostic process that initiates medical treatment for asthma is less clear-cut than that for diabetes. There is no definitive test that can indicate what to expect, leaving ample room for misdiagnosis. Mothers in this study told of physicians who they believed were hesitant to label and treat asthma at first, even when the parent was desperately concerned about a child's or baby's breathlessness. "Bronchitis" rather than "asthma" was the label sometimes attached to early outbreaks. As a result of this evasion, the undiagnosed child did not come under immediate treatment or control of environmental factors. In turn, some parents refused to accept an accurate early diagnosis of asthma—a tendency to denial less characteristic of diabetes, based on our interviews with parents. One mother, herself a childhood asthmatic, recalled that her parents had long before doubted her own childhood asthma, paying attention only when she passed out or changed color. Perhaps her parents were "ignorant," as she supposed, or perhaps they were like a few other parents I interviewed who said they did not want to think of their child as a "hypochondriac" or a "wimp." In a society that underestimates the significance of asthma for children's lives, some children at first go without full, immediate help.

Even after a child's diagnosis of asthma had been given and accepted, the situation can be hard to definitively pinpoint and track. There is no parent training, as occurs in diabetes while the child is hospitalized. Lacking systematic hospitalization and training, there is no family rite of passage to prepare parental caretakers socially and emotionally for their new palliative role. The lack of training or role preparation is strikingly problematic, given that the parental role is not easy, due to the stealthy impact of asthma.

Parents, through keeping day-to-day records, confided to me their relentless efforts to understand a child's strangled breathing. (See Appendix A for more information on parental field notes.) Parents' self-reports documented the strain to identify the causative triggers for their child's asthma, to correctly implement a complex plan involving many medications, and to take appropriate preventive action, such as installing air-conditioning or removing pets.[16] One mother in her daily records speculated, on various days, that her child's asthma might be triggered by dampness, the food additive MSG, cats (with which her son nevertheless played), urban air, or cold weather. In the end, it seemed futile to try to isolate a factor.

To illustrate the challenge and frustration of managing childhood asthma, consider a partial record from Mrs. Brian, mother of Spencer, age six. Her records reveal unrelenting efforts to make sense of symptoms and ultimately show how she resorted to treatments other than conventional biomedicine, such as alfalfa tablets, since control over asthma seemed so elusive through conventional medicine.

JULY–AUGUST 1995

JULY 4

We had a cloud burst this morning during the parade. It started to get very humid for a while, and that's when it started. We gave him his liquid Ventolin, hoping it would cure his asthma, but by nighttime, he needed to use his inhaler.

JULY 20

He was up a lot during the night coughing. He came into my room, telling me he had a hard time breathing. I gave him some Poly-histine and he used his inhaler. We had to close the windows in his room and put the air-cleaner on. This was a shame because this was one of the first nights it was cool enough to sleep without the air-conditioner. I was surprised he didn't have an asthma attack during the heat-wave. It all came on two days after.

Note: We have a new dog. It has been a week and a half now, and I don't know if this is aggravating his allergies. We have never noted any symptoms before when he was around dogs.

AUGUST 1

We have decided to start him on some vitamin therapies. We've been doing some looking into, and have found that taking alfalfa tablets will help. This is to be used as a preventative, not as a substitute for his other meds. We're working on the theory—can't hurt—might help?

AUGUST 2

We decided that five tablets of alfalfa in the AM and five tablets at PM should be fine. He also doesn't seem to mind taking a few other vitamins. . . . The true test will be in the fall when the mold count gets higher. We've had rather dry weather which is good for him, bad for the grass (just kidding).

AUGUST 15
Still taking all the vitamins and alfalfa. We even had a trip to
Antioch (Illinois). That's where his grandmother lives. She has
two small ponds in her backyard, and is surrounded by forest.
Spencer wasn't bothered at all by the pond. We thought he
might have a reaction to all the pollen and mold there is by the
forest. We don't know if it's the alfalfa helping, or the mold
count there was very low.

AUGUST 19
I received a letter in the mail today regarding his asthma from
the school nurse. She wondered if he needed regular preventative medicine or just an inhaler when needed. I told her only
when needed, and we weren't sure how much of his asthma
was exercise induced. She told us she would keep a special
lookout for us after Spencer had gym class or recess.

When school started, ten days after the August 19 entry, Mrs. Brian
made eight additional entries, all concerning the ups and downs of
her son's asthma, what might have caused it, and how it was being
treated (through pharmaceuticals, as well as vitamins and alfalfa).
Yet despite this monitoring and systematic reflection, the factors
she observed refused to provide a coherent understanding of how
they interacted to cause asthma. And her hypotheses left out potentially crucial factors. Despite her son's improvement when visiting his grandmother's house, Mrs. Brian did not consider the
issue of environmental tobacco smoke and continued to smoke
at home. She also did not weigh the preventive advantage of air-
conditioning, even though her son's condition improved during a
heat wave when the air-conditioner was used. She did puzzle over
another issue: the new family pet, a dog. But the allergic potential
of the dog seemed to be considered only after the dog was already
part of the family. Overall, Mrs. Brian's reasoning focused more on
scanning for and picking out problems, less on means of prevention. Given that some problems occurred continuously, including

secondhand cigarette smoke, the family erred in its process of elimination, as some familiar and pervasive aspects of Spencer's world were ignored.

In contrast to mothers of diabetic children who deftly juggled food, exercise, and insulin to control diabetes, this caring mother of an asthmatic child fumbled as she tried to put straight the tangled factors involved in asthma. Not present was the diabetic parent's deft monitoring and commitment to prevention, aided by tools that could accurately weigh and measure the controllable elements. The parental struggle with asthma carries less definitive control, leaving greater room for error and futility. The causative components can include far-reaching atmospheric factors (weather, mold count, pollution, etc.), and yet these factors are so omnipresent and insubstantial that they, in effect, vanish into thin air. In the face of asthma, parents struggled with countless ever-present threats, some of which dwelled in the air right around them yet passed unrecognized. Asthma overwhelms one's capacity to explain it, through sheer pervasiveness and a complex of potential vaporous hazards.

Because asthma's causes are indeterminate, society has given rise to folk beliefs that seek to clarify matters otherwise obscure. One such folk belief is the widespread notion that children eventually grow out of asthma. Thinking that "he'll grow out of it" no doubt offers solace to an adult caring for, or witnessing, a gasping, strangling child. But the facts don't support the cultural notion; a return of symptoms is possible, even among the 50 percent of children whose symptoms abate by age fifteen. Severely asthmatic children like those I interviewed are generally known to have symptoms into adulthood.[17]

Another prevailing cultural belief is that asthma is a minor hindrance that does not kill anyone. Complacency is thereby given sanction. Although deaths occur in a minority of asthma cases, hundreds of children do die of the condition each year, in contrast to this cultural presupposition. And death rates are increasing, often because of insufficient medical attention.[18] Asthma, like driving, can be deadly if it is mismanaged. Several children in this study volunteered, without probing, that they were personally familiar with a relative or adult neighbor who had died during an asthma attack. The inability to breathe freely, from the patient's perspective, carries potent meaning: It reminds the sufferer that death is possible.

Thus asthma is not dismissible as "minor" or temporary, in the eyes of its young victims. For the afflicted child, impeded breathing bears with it a felt risk to comfort, well-being, and survival. Children, mincing no words, described asthmatic breathing as an experience uncomfortably akin to suffocation. "I don't like having asthma feelings. It makes me feel like I'm gonna die," a seven-year-old commented. A six-year-old reasoned that "if you don't breathe you can die. If you hold your breath for a very long time." An eight-year-old drew a picture of himself when ill. "I'd be thinking I'd better get my inhaler fast and real quick," he described the scene. "Because if I run out of breath too long, I could die." To sufferers, the implications of poor breathing are obvious at a young age.

Asthma as Children Define It

What is that a picture of? It looks like a picture I saw at my doctor's. Is it the heart, or the liver? Is it something in the stomach? I don't know if there's any asthma in that picture. It looks kind of like a tree I guess. I know what asthma means, it means your breathing is clogged up and you have to take medicine. But I don't know about that picture you're showing me.

That's a picture of the lungs, and those are the tubes you use to breathe. Did you forget that?

Despite their awareness of the importance of breathing to life, most five- to eight-year-old informants with asthma did not understand asthma in terms of biomedical principles. Notions about airways, inflammation, and that invisible, inchoate substance, oxygen, didn't enter into most children's discourse. Instead, as was true for children with diabetes, it was the familiar regimen of medical intervention that was most salient to young children. Inhalers, spacers, and nebulizers, which visibly serve to aid breathing, are vivid signals for them of regained control and of asthma itself.[19] In other words, the concrete daily events of treating asthma and its symptoms defined asthma for children, rather than the biomedically defined disease. Among children exposed to educational materials that emphasized the disease process and involved physical organs, such as those shown at summer camp or at a physician's office, most generally did not treat the information as highly salient; their indifference supports the idea that children conceive of asthma in ways other than as a biomedical construct. One boy used the term "asthma" to designate his metered-dose inhaler, linguistically equating the treatment with the illness. When I asked children to explain what happens during asthma, their responses mainly left out biomedical notions of the disease process. In the following conversation with Sally, age eight, my queries about asthma met with direct avoidance.

> CDC: Before we start, I want to make sure I understand one important thing. What is asthma?
> SALLY: Hmm. [Laughs]
> CDC: What do you think?
> SALLY: That's hard. . . . How should I know? I'm in third grade. . . . How should I know?

Many other children, when asked to define asthma, focused on their personally felt symptoms, not the biomedical process, as did five-year-old Nate.

CDC: What is asthma, anyway? What do you think it is?
NATE: It affects your breathing. And that's what I think
of it. . . . I start breathing really slow [and] my air gets all
clogged up.

Defining asthma in terms of the medical paraphernalia
of treatment was especially common and is similar to the way
in which diabetic children defined their illness through treatment
procedures (see Chapter 2). Young asthma sufferers had a thorough, tangible familiarity with devices like inhalers, spacers, and
nebulizers. Invited to explain what was happening to a doll imagined to have asthma, a six-year-old boy said, "She had been coughing a lot and needs, like, spray machines." A five-year-old girl
explained that she could tell if a place was an "asthma place" based
on whether or not there was an Inspirease spacer there. The treatment device, in this case the spacer, served as a palpable indicator of asthma. Another girl, age seven, volunteered that using
her inhaler was how she could tell when she was sick with
asthma: "I'm not sick if I don't do my inhaler." A six-year-old boy
perceived the treatment device as central; when he was asked,
"What happens when you have asthma?" he readily declared,
"I have to get my nebulizer." No mention of his body or its processes needed to be made. In children's everyday understanding,
asthma is generally a matter of symptoms met with concrete medical treatment.

Only rarely did an exception emerge. An eight-year-old boy,
one of the oldest children interviewed, had begun to internalize
the biomedical model of asthma and was able to identify and explain the role of the lungs and bronchial tubes when shown a medical drawing, unlike other children shown the same drawing. This
child with severe asthma seemed to sustain a sense of rational
orderliness, even calming comfort, from his biomedical understanding; he had learned how each of his prescribed medications

intervened biomedically in the asthmatic response. He seemed able to reason about his illness in a detached, somewhat analytical fashion. He might have been a poster child for scientific patient education had he not been so exceptional, contrasting with how most children interviewed understood asthma.

Even at the advanced age of ten and eleven, girls studied through participant observation at asthma camp tended to place salient emphasis on treatment devices for asthma, rather than on bodily organs or biomedical theory. For instance, the campers jointly invented an imaginary toy on the last day of camp, an "Asthma Barbie" doll, accessorized with an inhaler, nebulizer, and oxygen mask. Asthma Barbie would come with toy paraphernalia of treatment—her defining characteristic. One girl added that she would also like a "Surgery Barbie," a doll that could be opened up to look at her heart, lungs, and liver. But she planned to play with Surgery Barbie for general anatomical interest (by taking out all the organs and putting them back in order), not to play or enact asthma games. The Barbie doll with inhaler, nebulizer, and oxygen mask would be the more suitable choice to role-play asthma, this group of campers agreed.[20]

Psychological inquiry into children's conceptions of illness has built a strong case that children's notions do not reflect or even approach the biomedical understanding that prevails among adults.[21] In contrast to the rationalist disease model taken for granted by physicians, children's knowledge of illness has been described by investigators as more emotion laden. Children have been said to associate illness with a capricious source beyond individual control or explanation.[22] Children are better acquainted and involved with the consequences and treatment of illness, which affect them, than they are with its biomedical causes.

In recent years, developmental psychologists have come to regard children's everyday knowledge as formed of coherent "intuitive theories." Youthful theories for illness intuitively include much that is not biomedical.[23] Asthma, like a child's constitution of reality in general, occurs in a social context.[24] The social events of diabetes and asthma, the culture-derived (that is, medical) artifacts, and the respective emotional meanings largely supersede abstract biomedical explanations, even when biomedical notions have been presented to the child.[25]

Arthur Kleinman has encouraged medical practitioners to distinguish between the practitioner's narrow biological construction of disease, on the one hand, and the patient's broader sense of illness (replete with everyday ramifications and intuitions from personal experience), on the other hand.[26] Developing a sense of self and forming a nascent impression of the world in which they live, children are a particularly compelling case for Kleinman's emphasis on a patient's experience of illness. To understand asthma in children's lives, the young sufferers need to be understood in their own right. An Asthma Barbie based on biomedical notions likely would not sell (nor would it likely provide effective education about asthma) unless its features were to include what is salient to children: the treatments, which are crucial to children's own understandings of asthma. A strictly biomedical, conceptual take on asthma carries too little relevance in the face of children's direct, lived experience.[27]

Understanding children's daily social environments, and children's active roles in construing medical interventions and symptoms, provides a wider lens through which to view children's worlds. For children living with asthma, the apparatus of treatment forms a vivid part of their everyday milieu. So too does the recurrent troublesome breathing that challenges their sense of well-being. A paucity of breath, and a plenitude of treatment, constitute the experience of severe asthma for young children, if their version of truth be told.[28]

Medicinal Value

If I had a magic wand, all asthma medicine would taste good, not like the yucky stuff. And my inhaler and breathing machine would work as fast as I can snap my fingers, so I could start breathing and go and play. My breathing machine takes ten thousand years. That's how slow it seems to me. Sometimes, I play games with myself when I do my breathing machine. I pretend I have a friend who is a dragon, and the dragon breathes smoke. You know the steam coming from the machine? That's dragon smoke. Another game is, I have a toy airplane. I fly my airplane through the steam. I pretend to fly away, to a place away from this. That's really fun to pretend, getting up and away.

I don't remember how it got started, but she and I have always made a game out of taking her inhaler. She has to hold in her breath to the count of ten when she takes it. So I started counting for her while she did that, in funny ways, like the Count's voice on Sesame Street, or in Pig Latin, or even in other languages. I would be clapping my hands while we counted. It made the whole thing more fun for her. She always reminds me to count if I forget. When she has to sit to do her nebulizer, I sit too, and read her a story. She calls it the "happy happy joy joy" time, you know, like that saying on the TV show. I saved an extra mask from her nebulizer and she plays with it sometimes with her friends. She pretends she is the doctor, and her friend is the one with asthma. So then her friend wears the mask to pretend she's taking the nebulizer. "Just sit there, and if you're bored, you can have your mom read you a story," she tells her friend, as if it were doctor's orders. It makes it so much easier when there's some fun and TLC, you know—tender loving care—about the medicine.

The maxim that necessity is the mother of invention has its proof in the impressive imaginative strategies among children and parents who continually deal with asthma. Asthma is a formidable reality for a family; its symptoms can provoke life-and-death anxiety. An attack of asthma can bring nearly paralyzing fear, but play provides a way for the parent, the child, or both to escape or lighten the situation, if only through fantasy.

A child struck with uncontrollable breathlessness faces what Winnicott calls an impingement on personhood, a crisis of "being and annihilation." That is, asthma poses a fundamental psychic threat against which the child is essentially unshielded.[29] The notion that breathing is a given, and therefore that existence is a given, is contradicted when breathing falters. There is anxiety in this dilemma, both for child and parent. "Scared" was a word children often used in describing the feelings of asthma. For example, one child described asthma as a "scary" experience analogous to having a "bad guy" nearby. Another youngster said that in a place analogous to asthma, you had to say "bye-bye life." Asthma has ominous associations, as an experience "far from air" in which you "worry you might die."

Fear was described by mothers also, such as one who tearfully remembered her eight-year-old son's hospitalization and placement in an oxygen tent at the age of three. "That picture is still in my head. I could see me sitting in the front room, crying, with him hanging in my arms . . . with his head hanging over, just hanging back." She mimicked a limp head and neck. "I'll just never forget. And I'll never forget the two weeks of going back and forth, back and forth [to the hospital], and then telling me he has to go in the hospital again, and Why? We just don't understand. . . . Why can't you prevent something like this happening? . . . Gee God! Something could happen so—" Her voice trailed off. "Even when he's older, I'll never lose the fear."

In the grip of fear themselves, mothers felt ill prepared to deal with asthma's grip on their child. After standing by and witnessing a child struggling to breathe, the parent needed to regain a sense of control, just as did the child. And since asthma is chronic, the mortal threat and loss of control recurred over a series of successive, unpredictable attacks.

What could help? Medications gave at least a semblance of control, both in medical intent and in emotional reassurance. Medicines that provided immediate relief carried a tacit assurance of trust and safety, particularly for the child—bearing more emotional meaning than medicines taken for prevention.

Yet in the final reckoning, maternal trust in medicines has limits. Many parents were suspicious of the medicines their children take for asthma, due to worry that a remedy might be habit-forming, cause side effects, or otherwise present a secondary threat on top of asthma itself. Already anxious about asthma as a threat to her child, one mother explained that her anxiety was further entrenched after an unpleasant experience with medication. She gave her eight-year-old son an over-the-counter drug that interacted with a prescribed inhaled medicine, triggering a crisis that made her voice tremble upon retelling. "I gave him his Slo-bid and immediately afterwards gave him an over-the-counter decongestant. He sat in the corner and held his chest. And he said, 'Mom, my heart hurts.' And his heart is racing like this." She gestured rapid movement. "It scared the devil out of me . . . I gave two medications close together, and I called the doctor at three o'clock in the morning, and that to me is the ultimate sin, because doctors make you feel like—" She shook her head to show a physician's disapproval. "His heart was racing so fast. I didn't know whether I should take him to the hospital or leave him. And then they told me what to do, and I thought, I'm not doing it right. . . . You have to take his pulse and find out how close the heartbeats are, and if they're getting close to the point where she said [to] take him to the emergency room. And that immediately makes me panic. You know, not panic, but it feels like I'm [panicking] inside. Those are situations [when] you don't want to have your child's life in your hands."

The drugs and paraphernalia of medical treatment elicited a double-edged attitude from parents. Parents widely suspected that the power to heal could also hold the power to harm, in asthma. This sometimes meant not cooperating with the full regimen prescribed. Clinical research reports a consistent finding that "noncompliance with the treatment approach" is a major cause for failed pharmacology in asthma.[30] (This contrasts with the trusted and accepted insulin treatments for diabetes.) Asthma, an illness fraught with fear, is all the more disturbing to parents, who worry that the source of safe control may itself prove unsafe.

Nevertheless, asthma remedies carried reassuring meaning to children. The sheer experience of gaining breathing relief from a medicine earned loyal appreciation from a child. And when the medication was surrounded by a playful ritual, such as imaginative imagery and play during treatment, medicine held particular meaning for the child. Medicine can provide emotional, as well as physical, reassurance, consistent with the experience of children with diabetes. The emotional value of treatment to children is worth considering with respect to three modes of treatment: the nebulizer, the metered-dose inhaler (and spacer), and the peak-flow meter.

The Nebulizer

A nebulizer is a machine that dispenses medication to the lungs. It does this more slowly than would an injection or pill. Although not literally an iron lung, the "breathing machine" (or, as children often refer to it, "the machine") is a device to which a child is connected via a hose and face mask or mouthpiece. The child must remain sedentary and breathe through the face mask for ten to fifteen minutes or more while the full dose of medication is nebu-lized. Because of the air tube that extends from the patient and at-taches to the nebulizer, the patient cannot move around freely. The experience of being tethered or leashed to the nebulizer dur-ing treatment was a sore subject for young asthma sufferers. A playmate of one of the study children who himself had asthma agreed with my interviewee that the nebulizer was effective but boring. "It's a good thing, but I just hate to keep on breathing, breathing, breathing," he volunteered. Another boy compared a nebulizer treatment to lying prone in the hospital attached to a "breathing machine." "I feel like I'm locked up in a cage," he de-clared. Playing with a doll that looked like Burt (a character on *Sesame Street*), another boy imagined how Burt would feel during nebulizer treatments if he had asthma.

> CDC: If Burt's doing this, does he like it or not really? What do you think?
> BOY (age six): Not really, cause Ernie [Burt's sidekick on *Sesame Street*] gets to play.

Many children watched television during nebulizer treat-ments, although the noise of the nebulizer could make it difficult to hear the broadcast. Some children complained about medi-cation inhaled in mist form that it tasted bad, made them too jit-tery, or felt uncomfortable when sprayed into the throat. The mask could also feel uncomfortable. At least one child recalled being frightened of the mask the first time a nurse placed it over his nose and mouth. (Asthma, of course, carries a threat of blocked breath-ing, a sensation echoed when "blocking" the face with the mask.)

Most mothers agreed that it could be difficult to motivate a child to sit still for the full nebulizer treatment, since children pre-fer to be active. A case in point is this mother's lament over having to begin nebulizer treatments again with her eight-year-old son, after a hiatus.

MOTHER: Now that he hasn't been using that nebulizer very much, it's tough to get him on. It's tough to get him back on the machine.

BOY: I never go on it anymore.

MOTHER: It's tough. It's a fight.

A handful of parents applied ingenuity to nebulizer use, transforming this time into "quality time" in which parent and child shared a pastime together. The child might sit on the parent's lap for a story, snuggling close. "Just until the end of one more chapter," Mrs. Parker would plead with her bored child during such a reading session. Mrs. Parker also made up a game to link the storybook reading to the treatment: In order to turn to the next page, the child had to breathe in from the nebulizer. In another family, the parent let the child have a break to "stretch" in the middle of the nebulizer treatment. Such parental ingenuity countered the dullness of the nebulizer session. Children appreciated the diversions.

Operating a nebulizer was not considered an easy task, in terms of the mechanics of hooking up the tubing and mask, inserting the liquid medication, plugging in the machine, and turning it on. Nevertheless, a few children, some as young as five, knew how to do this entire process and demonstrated it to me. It was not unknown for a child to wake up in the night unable to breathe, prepared to operate the nebulizer alone in order not to wake a parent. In the end, no matter how boring the treatment, a nebulizer was a machine children counted on to "give you air" or, as one seven-year-old said, to "suck out your asthma air."

As a corrective, a nebulizer was considered by parents the "heavy artillery" that worked for severe attacks, to quote one mother. A nebulizer could restore comfort and safety and, as mothers knew, could prevent the trauma of hospitalization or a trip to the emergency room. Children complained about the monotony, but mothers recalled episodes of dramatic, severe asthma that had retreated, thanks to the nebulizer.

Photographs taken by families as part of the study sometimes provided vivid depictions of the nebulizer's transforming impact. One photo showed a "before" picture in which the boy's face was lifeless and pallid, with deep circles under his eyes. After the treatment, an "after" photo showed the child peacefully asleep, breathing well enough to rest from the exhaustion of not being able to breathe. Parent and child could both breathe more easily in an emotional sense, having put the tense crisis at bay, at least for now.

Childen appreciate the nebulizer, despite the boredom. In the MST (Metaphor Sort Technique) sorting, children compared the nebulizer to positive or saving objects, such as a rainbow ("It saves me so I can breathe better"), a bicycle helmet ("It protects you"), or an umbrella ("You won't get wet, just like [the nebulizer] gives you air so you won't die"). One child likened the feeling of safety from a nebulizer to a birthday cake ("You feel safe, like on your birthday with your friends around"). The nebulizer was befriended ("like a friend to you") or trusted (comparable to a teddy bear).[31] But it was not perceived as an outright "happy" possession, because of the boredom imposed when using it. A nebulizer, one boy said, was like a school bus that passed the same scenes every day and took so long that "I may be late for school." Time dragged for him while hooked to the nebulizer. In short, the nebulizer was a mixed blessing, a means of rescue but with tedium.

Medical anthropologist Gay Becker has shown that personal disruptions, of which asthma is an example, prompt an effort to make sense of experience and to restore order and normalcy.[32] Once breathing is restored in an asthma attack, and the worse fears prove unrealized, somehow child and mother need to navigate their way back from the brink of terrible possibility. The nebulizer not only provides relief from breathing distress, but also serves as a vehicle for transformation to normalcy for child and mother alike. Any medicine can hold a range of meanings.[33] A nebulizer, insofar as children associate it with "staying alive," has reassuring, restorative meaning. In symbolic terms, the nebulizer is an anchor of relief amidst the turbulent anxiety of severe asthma. Still, since the nebulizer inhibits freedom of physical movement when used, it is also an anchor that takes away the child's usual freedom. Nebulizers ensure that children survive, but for the time being destroy their full liberty.

The Metered-dose Inhaler

Alan Prout, a sociologist who studied the metered-dose inhaler, has argued for an inextricable link between human and technological aspects of illness. "This device does not simply 'impact' on the social relations of sickness . . . but . . . in using the device children and parents are enrolled into an ongoing interaction in which technologies and people mutually constitute each other."[34] In other words, the technologies used to treat illness become intertwined in the social process by which people interact with and influence each other.

Used in the social context of family life, the inhaler serves to keep life "ordinary" when children have moderate asthma, Prout and his colleagues have found in their ethnographic research. In Prout's investigation, mothers of children with moderate asthma tended to see their child's condition as a minor or insignificant matter. They paid only slight attention to nonmedicinal preventive measures, since measures such as eliminating pets, soft toys, and other environmental triggers would be disruptive of social relationships. Yet they gave medicine delivered by a single-dose inhaler great importance. Inhalers were convenient, quick acting, and very effective, which allowed a family to minimize disruptions to family life from the child's asthma. At the same time, other, more preventive approaches—such as identifying triggers, taking precautionary measures, monitoring with peak-flow meters, or making routine clinic visits—were relatively little emphasized. Inhalers caused little intrusion in a family's normative routine and allowed asthma to be viewed as a "non-problem." The breath-actuated inhaler is unobtrusive in its small size, its easy use, and its portability and yet, for the children Prout studied, was highly effective at minimizing the intrusion of asthma. Inhalers were a charmlike means of maintaining ordinariness among families of moderate asthmatics.[35]

Among the families of the children with severe asthma I studied, the metered-dose inhaler was seldom the only form of treatment needed but just one of many technological utensils. Among children with severe asthma, young children typically used a spacer device attached to their inhaler, which involved an extra step to enhance effectiveness. The spacer required the child to inhale at a deliberate pace. If the child inhaled too hastily, the spacer made a noise, a signal to slow down.

One brand of spacer, Inspirease, had an accordion-like structure that expanded and contracted with breathing. Children delighted in this powder-blue spacer; in some cases they inhaled and exhaled so vigorously as to unintentionally tear part of the plastic, requiring replacement of the spacer device. "You get to blow in it," said one seven-year-old girl. "You suck the air up like it's some kind of game or something." One boy who received bubbles to play with on his eighth birthday said in a gleeful voice that blowing through his spacer reminded him of playing with bubbles.

Youngsters liked to inhale hard through the spacer, since they liked to make and hear the noise it would emit. Ironically, the noise was designed to be a disincentive for children, a "warning" that they were inhaling too quickly. But for children, making a sound with the spacer provided amusement, not disincentive. The mother of an eight-year-old boy said: "If he's in the kitchen doing it, he tries to get the dog in the face with it as it blows out. Sometimes I yell at him." Recreational noise-making and blowing were widespread, for Inspirease and other brand-name spacers. It follows, of course, that such products might benefit from being redesigned without an inherent reward, such as noise, for incorrect use.

Amused play with the inhaler and spacer raised children's opinions about inhaled medications. Children complained less and with less fervor about inhalers, in contrast to the "boring" nebulizer. Still, a few children lamented that they were embarrassed to use an inhaler in front of peers, which raised issues of social vulnerability. Some thought that it was hard to use an inhaler or resented the need to wait after each inhalation before puffing again. Another complaint was that the inhaler "tasted bad." But generally, the inhaler did not have the pronounced disadvantage of the nebulizer, given that it was quicker and less confining for the child.

As was true for the nebulizer, children understood that their inhalers had remedial benefit. "It opens my lungs so I can breathe," explained a six-year-old boy. This gave the medical device a strong emotional meaning and an implication of life-and-death importance. A girl, seven, said: "When you're getting medicine it helps you. Your lungs come back to life." In the words of an eight-year-old boy, the nebulizer could be considered a "life saver," since "it keeps you so you don't, like, die." (This was a generalized meaning attached to all inhalers, as children did not distinguish between types of dispensed medicine; they did not explicitly differentiate between short-acting bronchodilators and long-acting inhaled medications.)

Perhaps as befits a technology with life-sustaining meaning, a few youngsters speculated that something supernatural was involved in an inhaler. For instance, one girl fancied that the "asthma fairy" makes the inhalers for children. Another child imagined that the "magic" inherent in her human mother passed into the inhaler and then to her. The routinely familiar inhaler and spacer could take on fetish-like value, in the sense of being regarded with enchanted reverence.

When asked to choose objects with associated "feelings" similar to an inhaler in the MST sort, children's appreciation of the inhaler, often used with a spacer, was unmistakable. Safe and reassuring objects were compared to the inhaler. Chosen repeatedly was a life jacket, thought by one child to be like a "bulletproof vest" that "saves you." A life jacket, another child noted, prevents drowning and therefore "helps you breathe" like an inhaler. Warm mittens or socks also had a similar "caring" or "safe" meaning comparable to an inhaler's, as did a blanket, a baseball helmet, a car's seatbelt, an umbrella, and a "comfy" teddy bear. Magical objects were said to be comparable to the inhaler—underscoring the sense of supernatural power—including a magic carpet, a magic wand, Dorothy's red shoes from the film *The Wizard of Oz*. One child volunteered that her inhaler was akin to a reassuring sacred place, the Secret Garden, from the book and film of the same name.[36]

Children with severe asthma felt the inhaler maintained ordinariness at a profound level. They viewed asthma as a threat to life, and the inhaler as a way to restore safety and, in that sense, reestablish the ordinary. The inhaler was, then, extraordinary—as Prout's earlier study suggested, a "charm."

A bond of attachment between the child and the inhaler was common. One girl compared her relationship with the inhaler to the bond she would have with a pet. A pet, like an inhaler, would be loyal to the child—perhaps even capable of rescue. Like a pet, inhaled medicines would be ready, if not to play, at least to comfort.

At the asthma camp we studied, members of the medical staff sometimes changed a child's medication upon arrival to achieve better medical control. Such a well-intentioned change could backfire psychologically, no matter how appropriate biomedically. An upset camper deprived of a familiar, security-giving medicine (at a time when the security of home was now a memory) was not easy to comfort. It was as if a security blanket (a similar transitional object) had been taken from the camper. This case was recorded in camp field notes:

> JULY 23, 1995
> Getting her to give up her white inhaler, the Tilade, was hard. She said her doctor [at home] told her to take it. . . . She did give up her white and pink inhalers for the blue one though. She has a real worried look when we talk to her about her medicine. She doesn't know who to listen to. . . . She went along with it, but her security was clearly in the white inhaler. The [camp] doctor turned to me and said, "We could let her hold onto it. I know it gets to be their security."

It is perhaps no surprise that children who appreciate breathing for its life-giving power become attached to devices that remedy their airways. Medicines become metaphors for the illness experience, as Van Der Geest reminds us.[37] Intriguingly though, the same trusting bond does not seem to evolve in relationship to the peak-flow meter, which is a tool of assessment rather than relief.

The Peak-Flow Meter

It was striking to me how few children used a peak-flow meter or even recognized the peak-flow meter I brought to their home for use in play. Occasionally, a child had used a peak-flow meter at the doctor's office but did not have one at home. One family who owned a peak-flow meter did not know where it was the day I visited. Unlike the blood-testing devices that were a routine fixture in the homes of diabetic children, this tool used to monitor asthma was rarely in regular use.

To be sure, there was one mother who used the peak-flow meter to monitor the child's well-being at school, at sleepovers, or when considering the need to adjust medication levels. Another mother used it to confirm a child's claim of troubled breathing. But apart from exceptional cases, the potential of the peak-flow meter to reduce the guesswork in monitoring asthma was not recognized.

Clues as to why the peak-flow meter was so little used were apparent. First, some families had never been shown or prescribed a peak-flow meter. One five-year-old mistook the device for a thermometer, presumably an object more familiar to the child.

Second, there was a pronounced tendency for the peak-flow meter to be regarded by children as a challenge to do well, implying that a child should "feel bad" when not achieving maximum levels. Like the amusement park midway game in which the player uses a mallet to send the indicator upward to ring a gong, children expected that they should breathe into the mouthpiece and, through sheer effort, push the indicator to its absolute "best." Of course, asthmatic children predictably failed in this ambition and were thereby disappointed and defeated. The peak-flow meter was perceived as delivering bad news about one's prowess at breathing. Two boys recalled blowing into the peak-flow meter, after each boy's father did the same, feeling deflated and humiliated at their poor performance. Other children aspired to match a "normal" score from the chart given to them at the physician's office, at a time when their breathing was at best subnormal. The peak-flow meter came to signify a failure of respiratory competency, among boys and girls alike. It stood for failed achievement in a culture glorifying those who match or break records.

A mother with an eight-year-old son explained: "We haven't been religious about using that [peak-flow meter] only because ... the chart says this is what you're supposed to do." She pointed to the "normal" range of function on a chart. "It upsets him. . . . He was blowing so much that I thought he was going to pass out. He was blowing, blowing, and blowing. . . . He would keep taking breaths to see if he could do it. And it was like a competition thing. . . . Instead of just being able to say, 'Oh, these are the results, and this is why you have to take your medication,' it's 'Why can't I blow like that? Why can't I blow this much more?'" The ambition to attain a high peak flow was evident in comments during interviews. "I can't get it up high," said a five-year-old boy named Paul. "I'm supposed to try to get it higher." Paul explained that when the indicator didn't go up high, he feels "bad." Another boy the same age explained: "The thing goes up. You try to make it hit fifty."

Although I did not directly observe the training and explanation received about peak-flow measurement, it seems a likely possibility that some children were set up for failure through the directions they received. First, children remembered being coached to breathe hard in order to exhale at their peak, forming an unintentional association with "trying hard" and "doing your best." Coupled with the instruction to breathe hard, families often received a chart showing varied levels of performance, calibrated into ranges of red, yellow, and green. Children then tried to achieve the highest level, green, often not a realistic goal for them individually. Finally, the design of the meter, which allows children to see the indicator move in response to their effort, may also invite self-evaluation. One breathes hard into the meter and watches the indicator rise, a show of strength and effort visible to all, as in the amusement park games.

A couple of children, when sorting objects in the MST sort, likened the peak-flow meter to an object that involved blowing: blowing bubbles or blowing out the candles on a birthday cake. In contrast to the metered-dose inhaler, however, the exhalation into a peak-flow meter instilled far less involvement and trust. The use of the peak-flow meter as an early-warning system has not nearly achieved its full potential among these families for at least two reasons, both mediated by social conditions: a lack of awareness, and the futility associated with a "breathing contest" that asthmatic children can "win" only by cheating. Since a peak-flow reading could provide a visible standard to confirm a child's report of breathing, this seems unfortunate. Children's reports of breathlessness are not always believed by adults; their suffering due to asthma then goes unappreciated.

Untold Suffering

Once I was in a store with my mom, and I got asthma, and I couldn't breathe. I was looking down at some jewelry. When I started coughing, I looked up to find my mom, but she wasn't anyplace. I wanted to hurry to find her, but I couldn't move that fast because I couldn't breathe very well. Then my mom found me. And she had my medicine with her. After the medicine I could at least breathe a little. We went home and I had a cold, so I had to stay in bed for more than a whole week. At nighttime, I woke up coughing and I got scared when I couldn't breathe. Even when I went back to school, sometimes I had trouble breathing.

My daughter's teacher thinks she knows about asthma, but she doesn't. She thinks the dear child is faking it, to get attention, like when my daughter is crying and asking to go to the school nurse. Yesterday my daughter told her teacher she couldn't breathe very well; she wanted to go to the nurse's office. Do you know what her teacher said? She told the sweet child to just sit down and rest, she'd feel better. It was over an hour before she finally gave in and let the poor girl go to the office to get treated by the school nurse. People don't understand. Some of them think asthma is not real, that it comes from children's emotions. After all, they figure it's not cancer or anything, it's asthma.

In the day-to-day lifeworld of an asthmatic child, the breathlessness of asthma takes on meaning mediated by social interactions. Amidst common cultural notions that asthma is a minor condition, children find that adults don't consistently show compassion in the face of anxious breathlessness. Most adults lack personal experience with drowning, suffocation, or a severe asthma attack. Without direct experience, adults fail to appreciate fully how profoundly frightening asthma is for children. Asthma can terrify. Young children revealed as much to me through their play and talk.[38]

Mike, a seven-year-old boy who lived in a family with three asthmatic members, as well as a grandmother who used oxygen for emphysema, knew about the fears of asthma. He was blunt when informing me what asthma means to him: "You are really bad at breathing." Some time ago, Mike's family had decided to give away his dog, despite Mike's love of animals, as a control measure to improve his respiratory health. He took oral medicine daily and used an inhaler when his mom gave it to him. He liked his inhaler because it "gave more air" when he had trouble breathing. He also had a nebulizer—his "breathing machine"—which the family kept at the ready in the living room to treat severe flare-ups. Still, he explained, sometimes even his medications didn't give him enough air.

Presented with a series of pictures of places (used in the MST sort), Mike identified something in every picture that he thought would give him asthma. The dangers ranged from bushes (which caused asthma just by touching), to trees, to any kind of green vegetation (because "if I went to the woods over there, I would get asthma"). He singled out a picture of a dense crowd of people in a downtown setting, saying that the closed-in or "crowding feeling" reminded him of when his breathing gets "clogged up." He washed his hands twice during one of our hour-long interviews, concerned that he had touched his hamster or rabbit, and that this might trigger asthma. Mike's world was for him a hazardous place, able to set off asthma at any turn. Urban crowds, nature, and even pets made Mike wary and set him on guard.

When Mike showed me around his bedroom and pointed to

the bed he slept in, I asked him to talk more about his nighttime attacks.

> CDC: If you were lying in bed and you were having an asthma attack, what would you be thinking to yourself?
> MIKE: Well, I might die in my sleep or something. But I wouldn't get scared of it.
> CDC: What keeps you from—
> MIKE: [Interrupts] Because . . . if I would die in my sleep, I would die peacefully.
> CDC: Uh huh, so you really wouldn't be scared of it.
> MIKE: Uh huh. Because both, all three, of my grandpas died that way. . . . So I wouldn't be afraid to die that way.

Mike told me he expected to go to heaven, where there would be no sickness or asthma. He knew a prayer with words spelled out on a plaque on his bedroom wall. The prayer began: "Now I lay me down to sleep." Mike provided the rest of the words, not shown on the plaque but nevertheless internalized: "If I do not wake, I please hope that I will be sent to heaven."

In the final analysis, asthma intrudes upon the very assumption and process of aliveness. During a severe episode of asthma, all activity halts until the asthma is treated. Even though the child may urgently want to play, he likely cannot breathe well enough to do so. Breathing takes precedence. Children become observant about the physical cues they experience when breathing falters. If an attack is prolonged and carries ample respiratory distress, the youngster may have to explicitly concentrate on breathing, sitting in a forward-leaning or upright posture to more readily take in air. During the attack, the child may develop a headache. Coughing may be so intense as to trigger vomiting. The exertion involved in the effort to breathe can cause muscle soreness in the muscles used to breathe, felt to worsen as the attack persists.

If breathing fails, so does life—a fact children who have struggled to breathe do not miss, Mike included. Mike's calm attitude about mortality notwithstanding, other young sufferers were worried. Admittedly desperate to get their inhaler during an attack, they knew they needed relief since otherwise "you could die, quick." Raising the potential for terror was the unpredictability of what could trigger an attack. Attacks were common at night, under the cover of darkness, when parents and siblings were asleep in other rooms (although Mike shared a room with his brother). Parents sometimes were oblivious and continued sleeping during a child's attack, not able to hear the frenzied cacophony of coughing. Meanwhile, a few children, even some as young as five or six, would assemble their own nebulizer to gain medicinal relief on their own.

Based on juvenile accounts, a child in the midst of a nighttime asthma attack literally has to focus on where the next breath is coming from, a meditation unthinkable to healthy adults who breathe without effort or awareness. Children, on behalf of their own existence, took the initiative to regain breath and safety. One mother shared a narrative of her six-year-old son Charlie, who woke her during an asthmatic episode the night before the interview.

> MOTHER: If I hear him coughing, you sort of sleep, you know, very lightly, like, "Oh, this is gonna be a night where he's gonna need something?" And he had to shake me. "Wake up!"
> CDC: Do you think he always wakes you up when he needs you, or do you think he spends some time thinking that it might, you know, pass over?
> MOTHER: I don't think he spends the time thinking it might pass over. I think he spends the time thinking "Well, am I gonna be scared walking from my room to Mommy's room?"
> CDC: Oh, he doesn't like to leave his bedroom in the middle of the night.
> MOTHER: Mm hm. We have a fish tank in his room, and I'll leave the fish tank light on. But . . . my husband . . . turns it off. [Laughs.] And it was off.

CDC: There was no light in the hallway.
MOTHER: Yeah.

During our later, private conversation, Charlie himself did not recall the asthma attack that occurred the night before. He remembered "throwing up," but not any difficulty breathing. Like a victim of trauma suffering from denial and dissociation, the defining features of post-traumatic stress disorder, Charlie forgot the frightening episode of nighttime asthma afterward.[39] As is known from studies of children undergoing trauma, forgetting or repression can indicate the severity of a trauma's impact and should not be misinterpreted as a sign that the child has survived unscathed.[40]

Charlie's mother was unusually sensitive and observant of the degree of terror her son experienced from asthma. "I've had nightmares where I felt I was suffocating, [and] it's a terror," she sympathized. (In spite of Charlie's breathing problems, Charlie's mother continued to smoke cigarettes indoors, perhaps to address her own anxiety.)

Breathlessness can terrify, a truth long ago narrated by Edgar Allan Poe. Poe's own mother died of a breathing-related disorder, tuberculosis, a death Poe witnessed in early childhood.[41] He later conceived a character in the short story "Loss of Breath" who was horrified and feared himself dead in reaction to his breathlessness.[42]

Writer Tim Brookes, describing his own asthma attack, also testified to the terror of breathlessness, and the concerted effort to breathe, in asthma.[43]

> It was an eerie, vertiginous feeling. I was confronting the normally unexamined mechanics of staying alive, like the clock face turning and staring at the movement in its own case. What are the most vital functions? Breathing. Heart beat. Brain activity. Of these only breathing is at all voluntary. The cardiac pa-

tient, sensing the onset of arrest, can't will his heart back to its measured beat, soothing it down from a frightening erratic fibrillation; he can't rip open his chest and squeeze once a second, his life literally in his own hands. Only with breathing are we given the devil's option, the chance to keep ourselves going by force of will.

Efforts to breathe despite impairment, then, carry profound emotional power. The asthma sufferer at some level knows and responds to death's implicit threat through strain and willed-steady nerves. The struggle to inhale and exhale makes the fragility of life keenly clear. In asthma, the sufferer meditates on each effortful gasp, such that the unfixed, fleeting delicacy of life is thoroughly fixed in salience.

Children with severe asthma face a formidable truth: Each breath we take is not a given. In this thought, peril looms. The experience can lead to denial, numbing, and signs of helplessness—revealing that children and families are dealing with traumatic experience.[44] Just as soldiers in war or rape victims sometimes experience a constriction of action, family members of a severely asthmatic child may fall into a pattern of restricted awareness and action consistent with posttraumatic stress.

Despite the very young age of the children I studied, it is noteworthy that some, on occasion, did not announce their breathing difficulty to the adults around them but discreetly handled an attack unaided. Perhaps children sensed that they needed to downplay their distress, in order to maintain normal social interaction with adults. In a now classic ethnographic study, Myra Bluebond-Langner found that leukemic children concealed knowledge of their fatal prognosis (except from the researcher) for the sake of maintaining ordinary social engagement with adults. Leukemic children participated in this mutual pretense to avoid the taboo issue of death, maintaining an intact relationship through subterfuge.[45] A similar process occurs among the offspring of mothers who are incarcerated; the children often remain silent about their mother's imprisonment and their own grief in order to maintain any remaining available adult relationships.[46] Asthmatic children seem tacitly to know, subconsciously at times, that their own terror can be too much for the adults around them to handle. They may set the experience and terror aside out of a need to maintain mutual social roles with adults.

The writings of adult asthmatic Louise DeSalvo offer further insight about the reticence to discuss asthma-related fear openly. In a journal of her personal encounters with asthma, DeSalvo points out that the sufferer can gradually come to tolerate asthmatic symptoms, because the sufferer eventually forgets how "wellness" feels. "My inclination has been not to describe how severe and disabling my symptoms are, but, instead, to try to tolerate them. The truth is that I've forgotten what wellness feels like." Members of De Salvo's adult family became discernibly weary of hearing about her attacks. "When I was at my worst, and could only talk about how sick I was [with asthma] . . . I once calculated that the most any listener—husband, child, relative, close friend, distant acquaintance—could endure without changing the subject, was about thirty-five seconds," she noted.[47]

In a society that does not glorify suffering, especially in the young, children may have no ready audience eager to hear about their courage. Adults would prefer to assume their child is invincibly healthy, even if this involves some disregard. One mother agreed to our interview only because she was reassured in advance, by phone, that I would not tell her child "the percentage of deaths per year." This woman's mother-in-law felt that the best way to handle her grandchild's asthma was to "ignore it and it'll go away."

For their part, children with hampered breathing perceived asthma as life-threatening, regardless of attempts to censor or avert that notion. Yet some simply did not talk to adults about the terror of death, no matter how familiar to the child by close encounter.

Suffering Retold

Okay, lets play doctor. I'm the doctor and you're the sickie. Now take off all your clothes except your underwear, hold still, and I'll give you a shot. Okay, now sit quietly while I talk to your mother, okay?

I think it would make a world of difference if my daughter was asked about things, like at the doctor. Like if they pretended to listen to her, at least. Mostly, they listen to me, what I have to say. I can tell she likes it when people listen. She loves being interviewed. It's somebody paying attention to her. It's hard to believe, but I think she enjoys telling these things about asthma. Most of the time, nobody takes kids seriously. And a lot of adults take themselves way too seriously.

Clinical experience shows that children—no matter what the reason for their terror—often need to express distress following a trauma indirectly, through play or reenactment or perhaps through involvement in narratives, including fictional narratives.[48] Often, straightforward talk may not reveal a child's feelings as readily as enacted play or artistic expression, such as drawing or manipulating clay.[49] Knowing this, I came to each interview stocked with supplies for indirect showing and telling. I was prepared to "hear" whatever each child wanted to express.

Handed some paper and markers with which to draw, Adam, eight, lost no time. At once, he began to render a picture of himself at gym class after running a mile. He described his distress from exercise-induced asthma. Adam said he felt "tired." Indeed, he was tired in more than one respect. He was tired after running (and breathing poorly) but also weary because he expected to have asthma and take "all these medications" for "five to ten years." He expected to grow out of asthma (consistent with the popular lore) but in the meantime had already had more than enough of the illness.

Amy, a six-year-old, also set to work as soon as she was handed materials to draw. She drew herself holding a bouquet of flowers, with a round structure emanating from her mouth. She explained: "It's an air bubble and I'm coughing, and I feel, when I cough, like I'm gonna feel really bad. . . . I might throw up or something." On a recent night, she recalled, she slept next to a towel to catch any possible regurgitate, since she was coughing so hard. The flowers she drew in her hand were imagined to be a gift from her mother. "I like to imagine someone gave me flowers," Amy said, since this would help her to "feel better." Amy's drawing reflected her suffering (from nausea), but also the need and value of comfort through the socially meaningful act of getting flowers, which had not occurred outside her fantasy.

Through art and play, children communicated to me that asthma amounted to a pronounced affliction, not a minor hindrance. Children's accounts included themes of fear and the threat of death. Young informants gave every sign of communicating to me openly about the bitter truth of asthma.

Just as diabetic youngsters disliked shots more than some mothers realized, children with asthma endured trauma, repeated over time, that was more distressing than adults fully appreciated. Adults had incomplete knowledge of youngsters who suffered nighttime asthma symptoms while the rest of the family slept, unaware. Some children kept to themselves the full extent of their anxiety, perhaps as a way to maintain a normal relationship with parents, or perhaps for lack of a ready way to communicate their fear. Lack of knowledge by adults led some children to lack sensitive reassurance.[50]

Writing about physicians who treat asthma, Rich and Chalfen stated that "regardless of their level of training or experience, physicians who are not themselves patients cannot know the sense of helplessness experienced by a young person having an asthma exacerbation." Rich and Chalfen used a videotape made by an adolescent patient as a teaching tool to show physicians the girl's asthma attack. As powerless observers, medical care providers found it difficult to watch a young woman concentrating and working hard to breathe, eyes wide with fear.[51]

Trauma brings a sense of fragility. A child with asthma meets danger where ordinary people have no fears: in swimming-pool chlorine, in flowers, in hair spray, in perfume, in holiday greens, in summer days (of ozone alert), in brisk winter air, in unclean bedding, in cleaning supplies, in others' smoking, in homes with pets, in dusty Girl Scout campgrounds, or in moldy basements. Facing a threatening world in which asthma renders ordinary entities into triggering menaces, children cannot avoid constant risk. Asthma, like a terrorist stalker that comes unseen, unpredictable, and unrelenting, can make hazard and anxiety an emotional habit.[52] In sorting pictures to find places "that have the same feeling as asthma," children chose images of foreboding and danger (as was not the case for children with diabetes, sorting the same pictures).

If he were there, said a six-year-old boy of one scene: "I would get really sick. . . . I think I would feel so sick I would have to take the nebulizer two hundred times. This is barely . . . alive. This don't have any color, for sure. We would both have asthma"— referring to himself and the interviewer. "We'd be splitting up because we'd have to be finding a way out of that place." A seven-year-old boy said of another scene: "It seems like it's kind of a closed-in space that not much air can get into. And it's not that many cracks in the walls and windows. I think you would have a hard time breathing. [You'd be] wheezing a little bit. . . .

There's a little bit of life, and there's air outside, but it might have a hard time coming in, cause it's kind of like closed doors."

Another seven-year-old boy glanced at a parched scene of fire damage, explaining: "This picture, I know there's trees and plants in it, but it's actually the leaves and the grass that help me to breathe. There's not much of it. And there's not much rain to help the trees live or the grass live." I remarked that it seemed as if there was "less life around," to which he agreed. Even when looking at a tranquil pond scene, an eight-year-old girl said: "It looks like it has mold in the pond. . . . [I'd be] sick." Another girl, also eight, described a fire-filled scene: "It's a fire, and if I breathe in smoke, it'll make me very sick. That's all." Of a photo of a demolished house, a girl, six, said: "When I feel the house is blowing up, is when I'm coughing. And when I feel like the house is blowing up, I feel real bad." She likened the feeling to her experience "sometimes at the coal mine [exhibit] at the Museum of Science and Industry; I might cough at the explosion. . . . I thought the explosion would kill everyone." Lifeless or lightless scenes pervaded the MST sort, for asthma.

A boy of six said of a picture of a dark cave: "It gives me a feeling like if I'd been there and there's a lot of mold there, I would be coughing a lot and I wouldn't like it." Responding to the same picture, an eight-year-old boy said: "You're all alone, like it gives you the feeling of being kinda scared. Because when you have asthma, you don't like to be alone and being scared because you can't breathe. Right. And it's dark, and there's nothing living in there, and it's just not a fun place to be."

Asthma creates a world in which breath and life cannot be assumed, a place that carries shadowy traces of dread. Parents at times feel powerless against asthma's threat, and children in turn lack reassurance. Despite children's appreciation of the relief brought by the nebulizer or metered-dose inhaler, asthma can involve chronic reexposure to the same fears, over and over again.

Experts with clinical experience in post-disaster trauma have pointed out that fear can be counterproductive, since it can lead to temporary hysteria, loss of control, paralysis of action, or panic.[53] Feelings of anxiety and fear during a disaster can be pent-up through the process of repression or denial. Children, it has been shown, may have fewer successful coping mechanisms than adults for recovery from intense, unexpressed fears.[54] Children may not actively complain to their doctors or to their caregivers, but their implicit worries became readily apparent through playlike interview methods.

Children seemed to feel better to have a listening person with whom to share their fears, as happened during the research process. Children with asthma, like children with diabetes, appeared happy to have an outlet for sharing their feelings, through appropriate means, to a caring interviewer.[55] Children enjoyed talking about pictures, making drawings, and playing pretend games as means to express their feelings. The profound anxiety associated with chronic severe asthma was safely given voice, through play. Providing a safe, age-appropriate setting to express feelings about chronic illness held value for children, as any play therapist might have predicted.[56]

Families and Asthma

I have a kitty. I know it's bad for my asthma. See, here comes the kitty now. I like to pet it like this, and sometimes I kiss it. I have stuffed animals, too. My grandma sent the stuffed toys to me. She says I can sleep with them and play with them. The doctor says stuffed animals could give me asthma. I have to stay inside today. It's so hot today, I can't breathe that well to run around outside or go swimming. Do you know the boy that lives behind our house on the other block from me? He has asthma too, but I never played with him.

I don't think her asthma is nearly as bad as the neighbor boy's. He was in the hospital twice last winter. They had to get rid of their dog. He was allergic to it. I don't know how they handled the kids when the dog left. I never really talked to them about it.

Diabetic families as a group and asthmatic families as a group offer a study in contrasts. Based on this research, almost all the families with a diabetic child actively took part in an organized support group. Only one family with an asthmatic child had attempted (unsuccessfully) to attend or organize a support group of asthmatic parents and children.

A majority of the families with a diabetic child sent that child to a summer camp designed for children with the illness, such as a nearby diabetes camp organized by parents' grassroots efforts. None of the asthmatic children interviewed had ever been to a comparable "asthma camp." Many parents of asthmatic children had never heard of camps for youngsters with asthma, perhaps reflecting a lack of availability or promotion of asthma camps.

Commonplace among families with diabetic children was participation in a fund-raising activity, such as an annual walka-thon to raise funds for diabetes research. (Participating in the American Diabetes Association's "Walk for a Cure" myself, I can testify to the beaming, happy faces of youngsters whose cause was benefited that day.) No families of children with asthma had ever participated in a fund-raising effort, based on our conversations.

Families of diabetic children believed in the value of medical research. Parents and children often fantasized about the day diabetes might be cured, thanks to research efforts. No family with an asthmatic child fantasized about a cure; if any shared fantasy happened in asthmatic families, it was the fantasy that a particular child would be, in effect, self-curing by "growing out" of asthma.

In general, denial, repression, and avoidance were more characteristic of families with asthmatic children than of families with diabetic children. Many parents did not take full action to sustain a healthier environment for an asthmatic child, continuing to smoke or ignoring medical instructions to control environmental factors such as pets or household dust. In one household, the use of air-conditioning to control asthma was said to represent an act of "spoiling." This pattern of inaction is consistent with the findings of other investigations, showing upon visual inspection a concerning number of uncorrected risk factors in the homes of asthmatic children.[57] Despite the large number of children with asthma in the population, families with asthmatic children did not actively join forces with families they knew who shared their dilemma.[58] They did not exchange tips on how to manage the illness, in contrast to the extensive support networks among families managing diabetes. Nor did families with asthma organize into asthma-related social groups. With the exception of one family, families of asthmatic children did not actively seek to learn everything they could about asthma or to use that knowledge to combat the illness, as did families of diabetic children.[59]

In short, a kind of passivity or perhaps learned helplessness typified many families' experience of asthma. To be sure, this may reflect the difficulty of implementing asthma prevention, or it may reflect how families are educated or treated in the medical system. But to a striking degree, passivity was not nearly as characteristic among families of diabetic youth. Why such a contrast? Could the unequal level of initiative and action derive from the cultural interpretation of the two illnesses, that is, that diabetes is more dire? Is it related to the special trauma of breathlessness? Does it derive from the way each illness is treated medically?

Certainly, diabetes and asthma accrue different meanings in contemporary U.S. culture, even among those not affected. Diabetes is taken more seriously than asthma as an illness. Indeed, parents felt that others treated diabetes perhaps too seriously, such as a neighbor who wouldn't take on the "serious" responsibility of having a diabetic child stay overnight. The treatment involved in diabetes (injections and blood tests) is construed as intrusive and carries a stigma if done in a public place. Diabetes, in short, makes an impression on outsiders. Diabetes by and large is treated as an imposing, severe illness.

Asthma does not carry the same weight of cultural recognition. Asthma is not a "telethon" disease for which society raises funds for a cure, parents realize. Schools or teachers can be indifferent. "When the school just brushes it off as nothing, I get infuriated," one mother complained. "They invalidate the kid. The amount of time that [my child] feels the terror, it's like it's not important, it doesn't exist." Allergies and asthma are often subjects ridiculed or laughed at in movies or TV shows, as if mocking the sufferer's dilemma.

One mother shared a personal hypothesis that people want to "pretend asthma doesn't exist" as part of a cultural cycle of denial. That is, children with asthma (particularly the ones with severe asthma) provoke fears in others about whether the air we breathe can be assumed to sustain life. Under this assumption, children with asthma are like the canaries used by miners of yesteryear, when the birds' collapse indicated an impending air crisis. A child who needs an air purifier, spends days of high pollution indoors, or coughs in response to secondary cigarette smoke casts doubt over the air others also breathe, according to this line of reasoning. Much like people who live in the shadow of active volcanoes, most of us would prefer to assume that the air we breathe is a nonissue.

Victims of trauma are known to be silenced or avoided by others, as a way of socially skirting misfortune. Those who are close to trauma victims may feel the strain of stressed roles. Those who are intimately related may avoid discussing the trauma, with the best of intentions, to avoid a painful topic. Trauma can invite a "conspiracy of silence," despite caring and concern.[60]

The sight of a child unable to breathe carries unspeakable anxiety. Life begins with the first breath and ends when breathing does. Children's connection to life is only as reliable as inhaling and exhaling. Against this fact of life, asthma stalks, specterlike.

Reassurance

Asthma is like a mean vampire. It's scary and it sucks out your air. Asthma is the evil, grouchy bad guy. Superman is the good guy. He's strong. He can fly. Maybe he could invent a kind of air cleaner right inside of you, to keep the vampire out.

My daughter is brave, I suppose. But really, what choice does she have?

Physicians who treat asthma know that reassurance is crucial. Typical words of comfort, lifted from a doctor-authored mass-market book on asthma addressed to patients and families, are: "The goal of asthma therapy is to allow your child to live as normally as possible," and "Although asthma cannot be cured, it can be well managed."[61] Alongside such reassurances goes the common tenet that being well informed will lead to better asthma management.[62] As we have seen, however, a fully informed and empowered caretaker may be scarcer, in practice, than might be hoped.

For very young sufferers, who define asthma less in biomedical terms than do adults, reassurance takes its own form. Information not relevant to the concrete issues of children's life experience tends to go ignored.[63] Play, by contrast, is taken seriously by young sufferers. Play works as an outlet, because play accommodates the emotional issues involved in a flexible, creative manner. Psychotherapist Barbara Sourkes has written about the importance of play in ill children's coping and of its ironic power to have impact through, of all things, illusion: "The overwhelming nature of illness cannot be approached by reality alone. Paradoxically, the illusion afforded by play is what allows reality to be integrated. Through play, the child can advance and retreat, draw near and pull away from the intense core. These tentative forays allow the child to contain and master the experience."[64]

The "intense core" involved in asthma is tainted with dreadful possibilities. But children have resources of their own for confronting misfortune: play and imagination. They can bring their toy car to the emergency room and use it as a means of imagined escape. They can make a game of nebulizer or inhaler treatment. They can imagine that Batman is with them in the hospital, standing ready to press the call button to summon the nurse if needed.

The considerable possibilities of children's "imaginal coping" will be the topic of Chapter 4.

Imaginal Coping

Laughter is the best medicine.
ENGRAVING ON A SILVER PILL BOX

It is a fact that from their earliest years children live on
familiar terms with disrupting emotions, that fear and anxiety
are part of their everyday lives, that they continually cope
with frustration as best they can. And it is through fantasy
that children achieve catharsis.   **MAURICE SENDAK**

Knowing where the reality ends and the myth begins is not
necessarily the most important part of the story.
D. K. GROOVER

*I*n American society, we glorify the inventions of adults—computers, medicines, scientific theories—yet often trivialize the fanciful inventions of children. Imaginary companions have received bad reviews, for example, being decried as maladaptive or as indicative of psychological disturbance.[1] Adults also malign the tooth fairy, such as in the mocking expression, "If you believe that, you must also believe in the tooth fairy."[2] Wishing and other forms of magical thinking have been relatively neglected as modes of thought worthy of study.[3] Mere child's play is discounted, while rational adult pursuits are given greater weight.

An exceptional instance to the dismissal of fantasy lies in hospital-based child life programs. Hospitals increasingly have come to incorporate therapeutic play into children's treatment as part of child life services.[4] Child life specialists familiarize children with treatment, making regular use of play to aid the child psychologically. But not all hospitals have child life departments. Much of children's chronic illness experience takes place in the home, at school, around the neighborhood, or within the family, where play is not officially a tool of treatment.

At hospitals without programs sensitive to children's need for play and symbolic communication, problems can arise. Consider the experience of Grace, a seven-year-old diabetic, who told me about her hospitalization five years earlier as she drew an illustrative picture for me from memory. Prominent in Grace's picture was a very large tiger. The tiger was positioned next to Grace's "jail bed," as she referred to the hospital crib with bars. The tiger was in fact a stuffed toy, presented to her by her uncle when she was diagnosed with diabetes and hospitalized at age twenty-two months. The hospital scared Grace with its cagelike crib and hurtful procedures.

> GRACE: I hated lying in that bed . . . and I had a tiger. My un-
> cle . . . got it. It's like a huge tiger. . . . The nurses used to take
> it away because they thought it would scare me. But it didn't.
> [Sobs for several minutes.] And I was only two years old.
> CDC: How did the tiger make you feel?
> GRACE: It made me feel safe.
> CDC: Really? How come?
> GRACE: It kept me company.

Although the nurses thought the toy tiger frightened Grace, in fact the toy had been her helpmate, making her feel protected. The hospital, not the tiger, scared Grace intensely. Through a tragic misunderstanding, Grace's coping was misinterpreted and impeded by those caring for her. They took away her toy tiger just when she most needed it to face the hospital experience. A lack of understanding led to unnecessary emotional trauma, perhaps not an isolated circumstance across health care settings.

Grace had courage in envisioning her own protection through the toy tiger, a kind of transitional object. Children routinely muster such courage, very often without any aid from therapists or other adults, in coping with the hardships related to asthma or diabetes. This chapter examines the remarkable capacity of children for imaginal coping—coping through the use of imagination—and how imaginal coping aids their fortitude. My purpose here is to establish the importance of imaginal coping for children with chronic illness. The psychological and cultural mechanisms behind such coping, far-reaching and important topics to our understanding of psyche and culture, hold fundamental importance and merit further consideration in future work.

Coping

A child with asthma or diabetes faces exceptional circumstances due to coupled problems—the symptoms of disease and the vicissitudes of treatment. Medical intervention, although intended to restore normal functioning, has an adverse impact also, bringing restrictions, interruptions, and intrusions upon physical and social experience. Troubles arise apart from the symptoms treated, taking the shape of fear, distaste, pain (for example, the pain of injections), inconvenience, and boredom. Stresses that spring from the treatment as well as the disease become a part of the child's daily lifeworld.

Adding to the child's predicament are the distancing social reactions of others in response to the child's symptoms and treatment. Some playmates flinch upon witnessing diabetic blood tests. Coaches and gym teachers may bench a child using an inhaler to treat exercise-induced asthma. Squeamish relatives of children with diabetes are known to impulsively walk away during injections. Such acts of exclusion can "spoil identity," as Goffman so well explained.[5] As young as age seven or eight, some children in our study had already grown embarrassed to use an asthma inhaler in front of classmates.[6] In social interaction, children constructed a sense of self threaded with exceptionality—ironically, a stigma deriving partly from the very treatment procedures meant to re-store life to as normal as possible a condition. Children must cope, then, with social and taboolike consequences to their sense of self, derived from treatment as well as from the physical events of illness.

Research has documented that a supportive and well-functioning family can moderate the impact of chronic illness on young sufferers.[7] This study examined the supportive coping prac-tices that routinely surrounded and involved children, as evidenced by informants' photos and written reports, as well as during par-ticipant observation and interviews. Prominent among observed coping activities were play, ritual, story, humor, and prayer—forms of coping I include under the general category "imaginal coping." Through imaginal coping, a person engages imagination in coming to grips with circumstances that have real, stressful im-pact. (Insofar as prayer requires the engagement of imagination toward a legitimate sacred or spiritual realm, I consider prayer also a form of imaginal coping.)

Coping as a Process

The notion of imaginal coping is premised upon issues of mean-ing, as meaning is socially situated. Individuals engage with others and with cultural materials as they come to interpret the sig-nificance of illness. Within a family, shared activities of meaning making, such as storytelling or daily routines, sustain a shared set of values and understandings, as family members together make sense of suffering. Coping includes both knowledge (cognition) and feelings (affect). Meaning is mediated through a unity of think-ing, feeling, acting, and becoming. Thus, coping is integrated, ho-listic, and socially situated, rather than a solitary act.[8]

Coping takes place through the routine as well as the ex-traordinary social experiences of ill children. Coping may involve tacit levels of meaning that children do not necessarily articulate directly. That is, the contexts of meaning making may be implicit rather than explicitly stated or conscious.[9] Without intending to, parents or caretakers may hinder coping by such acts as taking away a stuffed animal, or they may encourage coping by providing a prop for play, a suggestion for a ritual, and so on. A parent or playmate may serve to co-construct a meaningful act of coping with a child, perhaps by devising or editing an act of play. For example, a parent might purchase medical toys and encourage the child to choose a stuffed animal upon which to "play doctor." The child may then choose to be a doctor who treats snakes (a veterinarian) and give mock injections to a toy snake, dramatizing courage in the act.

Even when play is routine and has no conscious rationale, play can advance a child's meaning making. Anna Freud and Dorothy Burlingham gave a psychiatric account in the book *War and Children* of Bertie, a small London boy and a victim of wartime bombing, who bombed his own bed with paper airplanes.[10] Bertie's play with paper planes was not consciously a way to cope with the trauma of bombing, and indeed it seemed to be impelled more than purposefully enacted.[11] Yet the paper airplanes carried meaning, pointing to the central traumatic dilemma, all the same.

At other times, children may engage in play with delight and openness, rather than consciously or explicitly to address suffering. As play therapists know, play is remarkable because it is not necessarily explicitly goal-oriented, yet it accomplishes profound outcomes. At the beach, for instance, a chronically ill child may become gleefully involved in a game of being buried in the sand by parents—and while the game seems just for fun, nevertheless the game may help the child to engage pertinent issues of control and surrender.

In the context of illness, coping is a *socially situated and symbolically mediated activity that addresses issues of problematic meaning*. Coping assists in the reframing of meaning, which illness is prone to disrupt. Coping, as the next section will illustrate, is a dynamic activity that occurs in a social context (even at summer camp), in which meanings are interactively shifted or transformed to achieve reconstructed meanings.

The Case of Illness Camp

Camps organized for children with illness have an impressive clinical track record. Research has widely found illness camps to be effective in improving children's control over symptoms.[12] In one such investigation, camp improved childhood asthma so markedly that it led to savings in health care costs of $2,014 per camper, through reduced hospitalization and other health care expenses.[13]

When children with a particular illness are brought together in a camp setting, they are typically exposed to adult-guided biomedical education about their illness, along with other activities; studies have presumed didactic education to be the pathway for the improvement in symptoms and control. Summarizing the effectiveness of a California asthma camp, a report stated that "the camp setting clearly is an excellent way for children to enhance their knowledge as well as to decrease secondary emotional/ behavioral problems."[14] Didactic knowledge was assumed to be a primary function of the camp and its main means of impact. This view reflects an intention that camp will transfer particular ways of thinking, especially biomedical knowledge frameworks, to the campers. In the attempt to teach principles of good treatment and promote adherence to treatment, camp personnel appeal to campers' cognitive knowledge.

A shadow of a doubt regarding the didactic function of camp derives from the work of folklore scholar Jay Mechling. In an essay titled "Children's Folklore in Residential Institutions," Mechling declared that a vibrant, resisting folk culture of residents coexists with the sponsoring adult culture in camps and other residential settings. He argued that children in camps are not passively social-ized by adult intentions, but that they resiliently use folklore gen-res (ranging from insults and jokes to illicit rituals) to occupy their own creative, expressive world. Mechling's view agrees with other scholars' work on children's peer culture, which describes play routines that embody imagination, improvisation, and covert vio-lations of adult norms—behaviors that enable children to appro-priate and negotiate meaning.[15] Straight, literal "teaching," then, is not necessarily the only, or even the major, source of children's shared knowing at camp. Mechling's observations deserve consid-eration in the light of our own work in three summer camps for chronically ill children.

Three investigators carried out participant observation while working at two camps for diabetes and one camp for asthma.[16] They were able to observe how campers interacted within each community, as well as how individuals paid attention to and made sense of the camp experience. They saw firsthand the process by which children reacted to the biomedical education and other ac-tivities at camp.

Young campers ignored, missed, or resisted a considerable part of the camp's biomedical education. That is, despite the best adult efforts to instill campers with biomedical knowledge about their disease, children paid less than full attention to their attempts. After one lesson at a diabetes camp for seven- and eight-year-olds, for example, some campers became restless, asking repeatedly, "When can we go home?" At a session about the long-term risks of diabetes, conducted while boys ages eight to twelve sat or lay down on their bunks, some of the boys fell asleep before the edu-cational session ended. Campers asked if they could play video games meant to be educational about diabetes next time, instead of hearing another lesson. But when the next day's lesson came, the boys' interest in the diabetes-related games did not last; they wanted to play indoor floor hockey instead, which the educator vetoed to moans and groans. Ignoring the veto, the boys played floor hockey anyway.

At the camp for children ages eight to twelve with asthma, the campers enjoyed some parts of the educational program, but their reception was not consistently positive. Straightforward verbal didactics did not rivet their attention or maximize their involvement, as field notes show.

> JULY 26, 1995
>
> [At] the medical education . . . [the] girls [in the cabin] were bored silly. They did answer, it was a lot of audience participation. . . . We had a picture of the windpipe, picture of the lungs, the nose, and little charts about what each one does, and what the mucus is to catch stuff in your nose, etc. etc. We also had bronchial tubes, bronchial was a word they made them repeat and think about it, and remember. Bronchial, bronchial, bronchial. . . . On the way back, I asked them what they thought of the education. Most of them thought it was pretty boring. Four of them said their doctor tells them all that stuff. Jill says she doesn't listen when the doctor tells that stuff [either]. . . . She figures her mom tells it better.

Education, it is well established, is anything but a passive transfer from teacher to learner. Learning involves the active engagement of the learner in some kind of involving interaction.[17] Learning does not simply pass from master to novice, in the way a house receives paint or a garden receives water. Unlike a garden or house, the novice can resist, misunderstand, or undermine the message. Boredom and sleep are just two ways in which learners can distance themselves from taught material.

Our investigation did not confirm the idea that the improved functioning of children attending camp happened mainly through didactic, biomedical education. As Mechling's work foretold, camp also provided a social and symbolic experience in which children created a separate realm of knowing. In this respect, camp was a backdrop for a unique social experience transformative in its own right.

Camp provided an opportunity for children to be with other children experiencing the same illness, so that the illness was "woven into the fabric of everyday life." [18] Children at camp shared the same medical condition and common treatments, which led to interactions related to issues of illness. For once, the children were not stigmatized in this social setting; here, their illness *defined* the standing social norm. Teasing about illness was pointless, since, as one camper pointed out, "Everyone is in the same boat as you." Non-diabetic siblings who attended diabetes day camp, in fact, perceptibly took on minority status. Siblings with unrestricted diets became the odd persons out, the deviants; an excerpt from field notes at a diabetes day camp illustrates the inverted status of healthy siblings.

> AUGUST 7, 1995
>
> Snack cards were handed out to all the children so that the children would receive the appropriate food groups for a snack [from the diabetic diet]. . . . The non-diabetic children either had "none" written on their cards or did not have a card. This caused some confusion, and a couple of upset kids when they thought they weren't going to get a snack.

In a social world where being chronically ill was the norm and eating a typical diet was marginalizing, social interactions took on changed potential. Idioculture formed, to use Gary Fine's term for the lore or culture of a variant social group set apart from the larger social universe.[19] Within the idioculture of camp, shared circumstances of illness were routine and communal. Illness-related behaviors constituted signs of belonging and were part of normal discourse. Diabetic children compared blood-sugar readings, looked at one another's ID bracelets, and kept a check on each other's well-being. Asthmatic children compared versions of inhalers, asked about each other's peak-flow readings, and kept track to see if someone seemed to be breathing too fast or wheezing.

Within camp's shared idioculture, children participated in joint playlike activities that reconstructed meanings not through didactic information alone, but largely through play. Play with peers, according to Lev Vygotsky, is the appearance on a shared social level of learning that will move to the intrapsychological or individual level.[20] In theory then, the gamelike shared activity of children at camp was on its way to constituting personal modes of thought or understanding. Meanings reconstructed in a peer group, that is, give way to personal meanings. If so, camp may well rework the meanings the children associated with treatments for illness, since treatments were often the topic of play for campers.

At diabetes camp, a favorite and happily remembered activity was creating visual art using syringes and paint, an activity that placed the medicinal syringe in the role of a fun, expressive medium. At asthma camp, an involving hands-on activity was using nebulizer machines to inflate balloons, thus reframing a medical device into light-hearted entertainment. Among asthmatic peers, playful use of spacer devices (usually used with inhalers, with a sound signal to indicate improper use) spread widely; spacers took on shared uses as intentional noisemakers or quasi-musical instruments, as the field notes show.

> JULY 25, 1995
> [Again today] there was a lot of play with the spacers. . . . Yesterday they were inhaling them fast just with the spacer, no medication [i.e. no inhaler inside] and making it whistle and laughing about it. Well, today they figured out how to do it with their nose. And so they were inhaling it with their nose and making the music. And that's 'cause we all have to stand around and wait for meds, and so they amuse themselves by playing with what they're holding, the Aerochamber [brand of spacer].

An innovative trick that diffused fadlike through the asthma camp's cabins was "cheating" on peak-flow tests. By holding one's thumb over the rear opening of the peak-flow meter, as one camper told and showed the next, a child could get a very high score, better than any nonasthmatic person could obtain. This was a gleefully satisfying trick to campers, to be able to propel the peak-flow indicator high without the frustration and self-criticism brought on by their usual low peak-flow readings. Peer culture taught campers to undercut the usual, "correct" ways of using devices.

Campers received prizes for distinctions such as having the neatest cabin or for winning at games. They especially liked prizes that were novelty versions of pervasive medical apparatus, such as a pencil case shaped like an inhaler, or a cup decorated with floating confetti in inhaler shapes. These prizes poked fun at familiar medical instruments, a joke appreciated by campers.

During the closing ritual at the overnight diabetes camp, to honor campers' fund-raising efforts before camp opened, the "kiss a pig" ceremony was held. A live pig, to be kissed by a human, represented the source of the insulin on which diabetic children depend, pigs. The pig is an animal at once repulsive yet life sustaining—an apt symbol for how children feel about insulin injections. The ceremony proved a meaningful rite for the campers, according to field notes.

JUNE 30, 1995

The main event this morning was "Kiss A Pig." All the campers and staff had raised money as pledges before they came. For each dollar they had raised, they could cast a vote for someone else to kiss a pig. The idea was to raise as much money as possible in order to vote the kissing privileges away from yourself. . . . Joan was runner-up so she got to hold the pig. Bill [a drug rep who came to camp as a counselor] won. . . . He applied lipstick and kissed the pig on the mouth for five full seconds, which left the whole camp in tears, they were laughing so hard.

By kissing the lowly swine whose food-obsessed species is responsible for insulin, participants in the kiss-a-pig event both applauded and mocked the significance of insulin. This was similar in impact to other camp lore that made light of wearisome medical paraphernalia, such as peak-flow meters or syringes, through playful uses. Camp idioculture produced transformative consequences upon meaning. Shared antics lightened the meaning of illness, poking fun at implements that caused suffering alongside relief. When ill children collectively made light of the medical implements that sustained their life, cathartic laughter prevailed. Mechling has observed, "No matter how deeply we folklorists probe into the most awful and alienating human situations, we usually find those humans able to make an artistic performance out of the little left to them." [21] All that the children needed to transform the meanings attached to their illness was a social setting, with its resultant camp idioculture, focused on their illness.

Campers laughed at their own vulnerabilities and dependency on medical interventions such as insulin or inhalers. Humor and fun reduced the tension over literally crying needs, allowing difficult issues to be reassessed and to some degree relieved. Theorists have argued that catharsis is made possible by an "aesthetically distanced" experience in which safety (through social support) and distress (not denial) both occur. [22] At camp, children were at a distance from home, forming a new community with others in similar straits. Denial was obfuscated in the company of other sufferers. Symbolism (poetically expressed through music played on a spacer, or art painted with a syringe) allowed them to put the topic of illness at a comfortable distance from the literal daily experience of asthma or diabetes. The shared lore of camp and its shared social support provided the "aesthetically distanced" raw material for catharsis. Together, children faced up to, even as they laughed at, hardships.

Thanks to a convened social group in which illness was normative, camp idioculture reflected an environment ripe for the children to reframe meaning about their illness. Children improvised about shared issues through playful acts.[23] Mutually enacted improvisations led to shared practices, some of which were tinged with illicitness, such as cheating at peak-flow measurements or blowing out music through the spacers. Children did not directly put into effect what the adults didactically taught but rather treated the activities at camp selectively and creatively. Active participation, creative improvisation, and engaged filtering or selectivity characterized the children's learning.[24]

Camp included some planned activities ripe for interactive improvisation. On the last night of asthma camp, a climactic event was a performance of skits written jointly by campers from each cabin. This activity explicitly set up a context for campers to interactively prepare a performance. A cabin of girls devised a skit that parodied the "Three Little Pigs" story. A featured character in their skit was a wolf afflicted with asthma. The girls' version of the three pigs story (which Bettelheim has interpreted as a tale in which planning and hard labor could defeat the most ferocious enemy) reflected their own particular concern: inadequate breathing.[25] In the campers' version, the wolf visited the homes of three pigs but was unable to blow down any house (in contrast to the original story) due to asthmatic coughing. When the skit was performed for the entire camp, prolonged and loud laughter occurred at the following plot element: The wolf had, upon measurement, a peak flow of fifty, too low by mature human terms to sustain life. Happily, the wolf was hospitalized, received a lung transplant, and ended by feeling good enough to "huff and puff and blow any house down." The skit dramatized the defeat of a ferocious enemy, bodily threatening even to a wolf: asthma. The performance enjoyed hearty and lengthy applause, as the play provided comic relief over an issue of deep anxiety (a fatally low peak flow) and its fantastic resolution.[26]

Children with asthma or diabetes appreciated camp itself more profoundly than the didactic information it imparted. Camp provided a unique field for transformative play and improvisation within a microculture of children who shared issues of meaning, such as how to interpret symptoms, treatments, anxieties, and suffering. With their stigma banished, children could put shared issues into play creatively and interactively. Such camps aid coping, then, and may lead to improvement in children's symptoms and control, not simply by adults' didactic instruction. Rather, the discourse of shared play functions to symbolically soften shared hardships and affects the ways children interpret their necessary regimens.

When I interviewed at their homes six- and seven-year-olds who had attended a day camp for diabetic children, they generally had forgotten what was covered in the camp's formal instruction, although they had been at the camp only a week or weeks earlier. Still, they happily and proudly wore their camp T-shirts weeks after returning home, as if showing off their special identity as members of the camp. Likewise, they enjoyed showing me photos of activities at camp such as swimming, painting with syringes, or sharing time with other campers. Camp had reached them on a level other than the downloading of information. Children found in the shared activities of camp a chance to render illness more lighthearted.

Robert Murphy, an anthropologist who wrote in *The Body Silent* about his experiences with spinal-cord paralysis, dictated a passage when paralyzed in which he compared physical paralysis to another, more common, affliction, what he called paralysis of meaning.

> The paralytic is, quite literally, a prisoner of the flesh, but most humans are convicts of sorts. We live within walls of our own making, staring up at life through bars thrown up by culture and annealed by our fears. This kind of thralldom to culture

turned rigidified and fetishized is more onerous than my own
somatic straightjacket, for it induces a mental paralysis, a still-
ing of thought. The captive mind misses the great opportunity . . . to free oneself of the restraints of culture, to stand
somewhat aloof from our milieu, and to refind a sense of what
and where we are. It is in this way that the paralytic—and all
of us—will find freedom within the contours of the mind and
in the transports of the imagination.[27]

In just this way, camp made available a condition aloof from
conventional routine, yet ripe for social collaboration. Campers
jointly used improvisation and play, without planning and without strict reliance on direct instruction, to free up their view of illness. Campers found freedom in the transports of the imagination.

Stories

Illness disrupts meaning, setting in motion a call for meaning-
enhancing narratives—especially stories told by the ill person to
others.[28] This need for story, which has been mainly studied
among adults, is characteristic of children as well. Whether or not
a child is healthy, stories of personal experience are essential and
constructive of a child's sense of self and world.[29] Told by the child
and by the child's parents, the personal experience stories of these
chronically ill children included tales about the onset of illness, as
well as the ups and downs of living with illness. During interviews,
mothers recounted stories about both dramatic and routine episodes of illness, including some narratives that the children could
also readily retell. Shared stories reflected and reinforced the family's co-constructed version of events. At times, the child and the
parent disagreed about the legitimate order and makeup of events,
raising points of dispute or clarification. Whether by agreement
or by negotiation, the stories of illness experience were mediated
within the family in an inherently social process.

Children made use of imaginative or fantasy stories as well—read, shown, or told to or by the ill child. Fantasy stories, such as the version of "Three Little Pigs" told at asthma camp, are not nonsense; such narratives are in the end crucial to children's sense making. Asthma camp participants reworked the story of the three pigs to foreground issues meaningful to them, by identifying with the depowered character who cannot huff and puff. Advocates of story reading to children argue that children also identify with the characters in written storybooks, making active use of written stories to achieve positive adaptation.[30] Stories are proven tools of identity used for the symbolic bootstrapping of self.

Fantasy stories can be potent raw material for children with issues to resolve. One intriguing example from another investigation involves a healthy two-year-old boy studied by Miller and colleagues. The boy retold the "Tale of Peter Rabbit" over a four-week period, while formulating, reconfiguring, and resolving issues inherent to the story that were relevant to his own world. Peter Rabbit's fictitious troubles in the garden turned on issues of rule violation, conflict, and fear; the boy retold the story in narrative variants, within which these troubles (which paralleled the boy's own emotional concerns) could be posed and in the end resolved.[31]

Bluebond-Langner's ethnography about children with leukemia contains an account of children using a fictional story as a means of resolution. Children in advanced stages of leukemia living in a hospital ward shared an interest in E. B. White's fictional tale *Charlotte's Web*. A boy with advanced leukemia asked Bluebond-Langner to read to him from *Charlotte's Web*, choosing a chapter about the death of the spider, Charlotte (a short-lived story character). In the chapter, Charlotte was "peaceful" as she discussed her outlook on life. "We're born, we live a little while, we die," Charlotte pondered. Charlotte further reflected upon the good things she would leave as legacies—a sac of her eggs, good deeds done, and the beautiful world. In the story, Charlotte the spider died, alone, the very day she peacefully assessed her life. The spider's death addressed issues of immanent importance to the young leukemia patient. It was on the very afternoon he asked Bluebond-Langner to read from *Charlotte's Web* that the boy requesting the story also died. Story assisted this child to make even this ultimate resolution.[32]

Healing calls not only for rational information, but also for an intact engagement of self, a process for which story has proven generative potential. Persons of all ages rely on story for meaning, be it through Bible stories, popular movies, or family reunion tales. Children who are growing amidst challenging, stressful circumstances are a ready audience for the right stories, since they have intense experiences of which they need to make sense. Story is a way to reflect upon the experience of illness and to construct significance and identity.[33]

Claims endorsing the therapeutic value of story have a long history. The influential clinical approach known as bibliotherapy has long assumed story's healing value.[34] Yet little is known about the mechanism for story's therapeutic effectiveness with children.[35] Better understood is the fact that fantasy stories allow children to choose a pretend narrative reflecting their own concerns, and to use that story for affective purposes, such as catharsis or the reintegration of past experiences.[36] Children use story improvisationally, as it suits their own meaning-making purposes.

Our research among children with asthma or diabetes directs attention to a particular facet of how stories "work" to help children cope—through identification or involvement with a main character. The children owned many toys of featured characters in a TV story or movie. Via possession of the toy, this main character in a sense entered the everyday world with the child, serving (if the child so chose) as a force comprised of pretense against miseries or challenges faced by the child. Characters used in this way included superheroes from TV shows such as *Power Rangers* or *Teenage*

Mutant Ninja Turtles, and sometimes other characters, such as Snoopy, the Pink Panther, Ren and Stimpy, Sylvester the Cat, or Taz the Tasmanian Devil. Such characters served as imaginary companions or as transitional objects—toys animated by a child's devotion and willing suspension of doubt.[37] Like the Nutcracker, the Velveteen Rabbit, or Winnie the Pooh, these were toys (usually with an extensive fictional biography provided by film or TV) that reached out from the frame of the toy-pretend world to engage the world of the child.[38]

Superhero representations, in particular, served as powerful companions to ill (often male) children in situations of felt vulnerability. A diabetic boy, Carl, took a toy version of the Power Rangers TV character White Ranger to the doctor's office for his checkup and lab test, privately imagining that the White Ranger also had diabetes. The toy was a form of moral support as a character known to be powerful; in Carl's words, "You can count on him." Having the White Ranger as a privately fantasized companion led to the worried boy's assumed protection, even when facing a physical exam. The paradox that seemingly underlies the character's value—that the White Ranger is powerful even though imagined to have diabetes—couples protection with illness. In Carl's imagination, illness and power were not mutually exclusive.

Peter, seven years old and a severe asthmatic since the age of three, also made use of superhero characters. I asked him to draw a picture of "the worst time you ever remember, with your asthma," and he set out to draw a picture of himself sick in bed. At first he drew his own face wearing a concerned frown. Then he added to his drawing the sheets on his bed, which happened to be decorated in TV characters, the Teenage Mutant Ninja Turtles. Upon drawing the Ninja Turtles on the sheets, Peter erased the frown and drew a smile upon his own face, instead. The Turtles on his sheets, as Peter visually recorded, brightened his mood. Peter had developed a fantasized relationship with the figures on his bed linen, much as other boys might love a teddy bear. (Peter's allergies precluded owning stuffed toys.)

Peter's imagined relationship with the Turtles was one he counted on when he felt sick or anxious. "I think about, like, they'd be real. And they, like, help me try to get rid of . . . stop being sick and everything. They come up and help me." How would they do this? "He would disguise himself and go to the doctor's office in a suit. He would go in a doctor's office and tell him what's the problem. And he'd say, 'I've got a real sick person at the house, and he needs your help because his mom doesn't know what to do, and we need your help.'"

Peter was anxious about becoming sick at night, alone in his room, unable to breathe and unable to get help. But he expected these superhero reptiles (mutant and physically anomalous) to be strong enough to protect and help him. "Nothing can harm 'em," Peter said of the Turtles, explaining that they would help someone with asthma but would never get asthma themselves.

The Teenage Mutant Ninja Turtle characters were treasured figures to several children. James, another boy with asthma, ritually wore clothing depicting the Ninja Turtles when he received his allergy shots at the physician's office. James preferred to get his shots while costumed in symbolic strength, as represented by a Ninja Turtle. The mother of another boy purchased a different Mutant Ninja Turtles toy character each week, when she went to the store to purchase diabetes supplies for her son. He liked to pretend that he gave a shot to each of these reptilian figures, an instance in which the boy reworked the meaning of injections: He was for once in control, and the reptilian heroes shared the status of getting injected. The Ninja Turtles were toys that accompanied children to the hospital, served as decorations on Band-Aids, and fulfilled a role as transitional objects that made children feel secure. The Turtles represented a fictional context that gave personal solace to a considerable number of children, especially boys.

Children borrowed distinctively personal meaning from these and other pop-culture figures.

A five-year-old with diabetes, Brian, engaged in imagined play with another animated TV character, which he drew in picture form, the animated character Pink Panther. Enacting events in pretend play, Brian showed me how he would give the Pink Panther an insulin injection. He claimed that the Pink Panther "has diabetes in real life." This assumption was based on the character's presumed behavior on TV: "On the Pink Panther show, somebody offered him food and he said, 'No thanks, I have diabetes.'" When I interviewed Brian's mother, she explained that she had obtained a handbook for diabetes in which the Pink Panther had a featured role. In the book the Pink Panther showed "how to give shots" and illustrated other skills of diabetes care. The Pink Panther—knowledgeable about diabetes lore—had become a fantasy companion for Brian relevant to his world.

Remarkably, very few educational books about diabetes engaged children in the same way that the Pink Panther became meaningful to Brian. When Brian faced and mulled over the problems of diabetes, soothed by the Pink Panther, he felt accompanied and safer.[39]

Theodore Sarbin has observed that self-narratives are socially situated and collaborative with others, including imagined others.[40] Since identity is shaped by social relationships, even imagined ones, a child's imaginings can contribute to an intact, defensible self—for example, a self less vulnerable and isolated in illness. Associating with a superhero not only provides a companion in the adventure of illness, but also implies that illness, strength, and heroism can coexist.

When stories aid chronically ill children, the child's active, flexible response gives power to the narrative or character. A story's literal text, even if illness related, does not automatically assure a receptive audience. The power lies in the child's response to the narrative, not simply the text itself.[41] An interpretation mean-ingful to the *child* fuels the engagement and appeal.

Symbolic material has the potential for multiple, even para-doxical interpretations. The child's interpretation can include layers of meaning and unfixed ways of inverting meaning—such as admiring Mutant Turtles for their exceptionality. If children sometimes surprise adults by identifying with unexpected heroes, Mutant Turtles included, this testifies to the active role of children in their own sense making of stories.

Mothers of diabetic children often said that they read about or showed videos about the illness to their children. Usually, these stories left little trace in children's recollections. One exception is notable: A few children did recall an educational video about dia-betes that employed the analogy of a teeter-totter to explain the needed balance of food, insulin, and exercise in diabetes. This video, entitled "It's Time to Learn About Diabetes," seemed to make effective explanatory use of a child-relevant teaching meta-phor, the teeter-totter.[42]

It seems likely that communicating about illness to children in books, media, and personal presentations can be substantially improved by taking account of children's reactions and ways of in-terpreting.[43] Taking into account how children perceive, react, and construct meaning could be crucial in constructing such materials to make the most impact on kids.

Play and Its Place

Theorist and master play therapist Erik Erikson formulated play in broad terms: "[Play is] the infantile form of the human propensity to create model situations in which aspects of the past are re-lived, the present re-presented and renewed, and the future anticipated." In other words, play enables the remodeling of our perceptions of past, present, and future experience. Through such remodeling, a child can recapitulate dread so as to regain hope. Doom can turn to confidence, through play. Play can allow a child to feel like a new being, free of destructive forces within and capable of fighting off adversity without. When peers and adults join in or recognize play, each can "help the playing child do what he cannot do alone." [44] In Erikson's conception, play involves more than straightforward knowledge, for it also calls on the considerable power of imagination. Play involves a depth of vision—including the capacity to see and experience what is immediately before the child, as well as the power to envision and believe in an alternative.

While there are useful and important notions of play that address its social significance,[45] cognitive importance,[46] and cultural variation,[47] Erikson's clinically derived ideas effectively map a theory of how these American children used play to cope with illness. Children with chronic illness do express and redress past and present experience in their play, and do conceive and act out preferable alternative scenarios. Parents, peers, and siblings are sometimes part of the chronically ill child's play. At the center of such play is a developing self living amidst discomfort, a self who must seek strength for the challenging experience still ahead.

The important role of play was apparent early in my research among diabetic and asthmatic children. Throughout the home visits and other observations, play permeated children's lives. Play was subtly present, at times even pervasive, in everyday activities.

Consider Tina, an eight-year-old with diabetes who, during our interview, drank her milk from a cup shaped like an ice cream cone with ersatz chocolate syrup decorating the plastic. Tina talked of a past event and drew it for me: Her mother was in the kitchen eating a chocolate chip cookie, while Tina looked on sadly. "I always feel bad because my mommy always does that [eats cookies]. I don't think it's fair." During our meeting, Tina was eating a lunch of permitted foods. But Tina imaginatively used her imagination and the cup's ice cream "disguise" to reconceive plain milk as a sweet confection. This was a simple form of playfully redressed experience that Tina enjoyed many times over.

Another instance of food-related play occurred among children who were part of a diabetic support group—a group of friends who liked to play the board game Candyland during parents' meetings. Normally, the local world of these diabetic players barred sweet indulgence, even at social gatherings. But children converted restriction into indulgence by moving through Candyland's indulgent fantasy world. Candyland is a rule-bound game, but while they played, the children appropriated the game board's candy-laden imagery for an imaginary free-for-all diet.

Some mothers of children with asthma adopted a Poppins-like strategy, allowing the child to have a wanted taste along with bad-tasting medicine (akin to the "spoonful of sugar that makes the medicine go down" from the P. L. Travers work *Mary Poppins*). A mother gave her daughter a sweet snack (a fruit roll-up) after each inhaler burst. A pill was served in sweet jelly, for another child. At work was a "play" of tastes in which one flavor dresses up in the disguise of the other. It is a simple form of play, within which both mother and child jointly reconstrue an unpleasant experience into a pleasing one.

Time and again, treatment was the privy to playful transformation. A hospital that gave its pediatric blood-testing machine the nickname "Herbie" and an endearing ability to "suck in your blood" won over one six-year-old boy. Herbie the machine, he asserted, had been the best part of his hospitalization. Giving the machine a name, the boy assessed, made it seem like the test hurt less.

A mother of an asthmatic boy insisted that this strategy should go further, that hospital procedures should be called upon to render each device playful and fun. She raised the example of the asthmatic child who is about to put on a mouth-enclosing oxygen mask yet is already anxious about blocked breathing. She suggested that the child not simply be masked, but be shown the mask and encouraged to imagine it in positive ways ("Does it look like it has eyes?") with an attitude that the mask "is going to be your friend." Had a child life specialist been involved with administering oxygen, this might have been a feasible improvisation, turning the scary breath-blocking oxygen mask into a "friend."

In sum, imaginal coping involves using the imagination to transform and reframe the hardships of illness. Imaginal coping among children ages five to eight appears to be both common and effective. Imaginal coping involves the creatively engaged child, infused with the Eriksonian power of play to transform past, present, and future experience. Imaginal coping is cloaked in symbolism derived from cultural artifacts, such as particular toys, games, or TV characters. Despite its widespread effectiveness, imaginal coping has been a relatively neglected part of investigations of coping.[48]

Adults can serve to either encourage or discourage imaginal coping. That is, adults around the child might scaffold or encourage playful coping by providing or permitting a particular toy, for instance. Conversely, they might try to eliminate such coping by removing or making fun of a child's special toy.

Randy Sikes had dealt with the stress of asthma for almost all of his five years. By now a veteran of chronic illness, Randy had been hospitalized for pneumonia in the first year of life, and eventually the ensuing "cold that wouldn't leave," as his mother described it, was diagnosed as asthma. Randy's parents moved from urban Chicago to a small town in Wisconsin while I was engaged in research with them. Randy's family was economically pressed. They moved to seek a lower cost of living and to improve chances for Mr. Sikes to find remunerative work. Randy's severe asthma persisted in both Illinois and Wisconsin, oblivious to the economic impact on a family without medical insurance. Randy used metered-dose inhalers and in Chicago went to his grandmother's house to borrow her plug-in nebulizer. (His maternal grandmother also had asthma.) He kept a duplicate inhaler at school in the nurse's office; Mrs. Sikes instructed Randy's teacher how to use the device if needed.

Mr. Sikes smoked cigarettes, a source of indoor pollution for which Mrs. Sikes had acquired a small room-sized portable air cleaner. The family owned a dog "with short hair," Mrs. Sikes pointed out in defense of the allergy risk. They had already given away a cat they previously owned, since Randy had a strong allergic response to it.

Mrs. Sikes recounted that from an early age, "as soon as he was walking," Randy had a special involvement with toy cars. He played with toy cars when he was ill. When I sat down with Randy to interview him about having asthma, he chose to begin our time together by running out of the room to retrieve his toy race car to show me.

> RANDY: I'll show you my [car], that I like to play with.
> CDC: Oh, you love that. Now do you play with that when you're sick, that car?
> RANDY: [Nodding] Mm hm. [Zooming car around] Vroom! Vroom!
> CDC: Let's say you're sick and you're pretending with that. What would you pretend with that big race car?
> RANDY: The ride in it!
> CDC: And ride where? Where would you ride to?
> RANDY: Chicago!
> CDC: To Chicago? Uh huh.
> RANDY: Mm hm. And every time we needed gas.

Through his toy car, Randy mentally transported himself out of the present setting to elsewhere, although his gasoline was in short supply. His mother kept field notes for the study over a course of months, which recorded how Randy relied on his car as a means of coping in times of suffering or fear. She documented the following event during a bout of breathing difficulty for Randy:

DECEMBER 6, 1994

It is very cold and damp, and Randy's breathing is not good. He was very restless and breathing hard when he was sleeping. He is still very pale and not looking himself. . . . When his breathing problems come and he is having an asthma attack he sometimes looks up to me with his big blue eyes with the dark rings around them, and asks me for his green race car. And I get it for him. He hugs it closely and falls asleep.

Randy had several race cars, all special to him. During interviews, he imputed magical qualities to each car as an object that, he insisted, "worked wonders." He volunteered that his race car could make bad medicine taste better. He claimed not to even feel a shot when his race car was with him. Mrs. Sikes confirmed that when Randy was allowed to hold his race car at the hospital emergency room, it calmed him, acting as a "godsend." Mrs. Sikes kept a race car on hand at all times, sending one to school in Randy's backpack, and keeping one in her actual car. She was sensitive to, and grateful for, Randy's reliance on the race car so that he could find calmness when he needed it. "The cars have gone through it all with him," she observed, in a voice that showed her credence and approval about Randy's play. Mrs. Sikes expected Randy to continue to have a race car "tucked away in the closet" even when he was old enough to marry.

Mrs. Sikes recalled barriers to Randy's play, in particular within the medical system. Randy was not allowed to have his entirely plastic car (or his mother) with him during an X-ray, even though the car might have comforted him about a procedure that made him anxious. On one occasion, a nurse had looked at her strangely when Randy brought the car along to the hospital. "What kind of parent are you? Normal kids have blankets or pillows or stuffed animals. You bring this kid to the hospital with a car?" Randy's mother got angry at the implied criticism and defended the car as an allergen-free toy that "makes him feel safe."

Despite maternal support for Randy's car play, then, not all medical personnel were equally supportive.

In spite of the skepticism and sterile-mindedness of medical technicians, Randy's automotive transitional object served him well. Like other children, Randy was a creative user of cultural symbols, having adopted a toy that fit his personal need for calming serenity.

Many children used a toy (and sometimes a pet) to cope with medical procedures, just as did Randy.[49] Teddy bears accompanied children to hospitals. Toy animals got hugged during blood tests or sat beside children during a shot. Children's imaginings about playthings were apt to vary widely, ranging from toy cars or airplanes to animals or superheroes, depending on the whims of the child. The individual child needed and took license, flexibly and freely incorporating cultural symbols. One diabetic child imagined the syringe to be a zebra; another saw it as a polar bear.

Biomedicine is largely construed as an objective, controlled science rather than as an art of interpretation. Like any claim that presumes understanding, this assumed objectivity has a narrowing impact on the constitution of knowledge by precluding or discounting other ways of knowing.[50] Toys, cartoons, or tales tend, in particular, to be disregarded.

Unintentionally, biomedicine can undermine imaginal coping, as when Randy's car was banished during X-ray, or when Grace's protective tiger was removed. Despite the meaning-mending powers of both placebos and play, like the placebo effect to which it is cousin, play exists on the margins of medical care.[51] To be sure, play is recognized and honored by play therapists or child life specialists. But children treated in many settings do not have such an advocate for their play.

Rick, a mature-looking eight-year-old who was an avid player of video games at the time I met him, recalled such an experience. Despite his savvy cool, Rick summoned to mind without probing the "yellow giraffe blanket," a blanket depicting yellow giraffes that he had used to comfort himself before his diagnosis with asthma at nine months. Under a physician's instructions, the blanket was declared a potential allergic trigger and removed. Rick proceeded to wake up at night with severe panic attacks, interpreted by the physician as "just airway obstruction," according to Rick's mother. Rick's mother eventually decided to return the blanket to the child, since his asthma symptoms had shown no improvement in its absence. Upon the return of the blanket, Rick's panic attacks subsided completely, an improvement his mother in retrospect attributed to the blanket's return.[52] At age eight, Rick still had asthma but no longer carried the blanket or slept with it. Still, he said, it gave him a good feeling to know the blanket was in the house.

Some children expressed appreciation to medical professionals who supported imaginal coping. For instance, Mike, age seven, recalled how a hospital nurse presented him with a teddy bear to take home, when he had been hospitalized upon diagnosis of diabetes four years earlier. Mike put the bear to use. Upon arriving home, Mike decided that the teddy bear had diabetes too and was in need of the same regimen of care as Mike. The bear obtained, with the help of Mike's mother, its own injection gear for pretend insulin shots. The bear had its own meter and lancet for pretend blood tests, performed by the child. Mike's mother explained that it had been up to Mike to decide whether the bear's blood-sugar reading was normal, high, or low. His mother felt that in this play, Mike had a chance to "be in control" of the bear's readings as an antidote to "being at the mercy" of his illness.

The director of a camp for eight- to twelve-year-old asthmatics also understood the power of play objects. She brought to camp two stuffed animals of her own: Ally Alligator and Monique. Monique was a dog, complete with a stand-up-by-itself leash. Both of these creatures had asthma, the director told the children, and she carried them everywhere to give kids a chance to stop and pet the chronically ill creatures. Ally and Monique presumably needed care and comfort, as the asthmatic children would expect of an animal with asthma. A homesick, anxious camper was given Monique to take care of for a day, and this had a remarkable cheering effect. The assignment to babysit for Monique "worked like a charm" to cure homesickness, according to the field notes kept by a counselor.

A cabin of ten-year-old girls actively pretended stories about the vulnerable Ally and Monique when asked to take charge of the creatures.

> JULY 28, 1995
> We played with them through lunch and made sure they were safe and took charge of them. . . . Ally swallowed a watermelon seed during lunch, and . . . Monique got a bee sting.

Later in the week at camp, Monique was secretly kidnapped, and the campers tirelessly searched for her. [Monique was later released by the kidnappers as part of a cabin's skit at the last night's camp performance.]

Clearly, these youngsters, who so totally depended upon mothers for care and were at camp temporarily motherless, thrived when asked to care for an imaginal asthmatic animal. The child designated to help gained by playing at being a caretaker. The power to take care was an empowering dimension of identity. Through play a child could incorporate caretaking as a dimension of capable selfhood.[53]

By providing resources for children's play, caretakers can choose to actively scaffold and support imaginal coping. If, however, imaginal coping is disregarded or eliminated, the severing can have unforeseen detrimental effects even years later. Recall the instances of Grace losing her tiger and Rick being deprived of his blanket—in both cases, the children reported grief years later. Medical treatment can disrupt an ongoing source of coping by denying access to an established routine. Play can serve to mediate the trauma of treatment, but only when caretakers are sensitive and supportive about the child's practices.[54]

Being sensitive to a child's attachments to playthings raises a thorny dilemma when the child has a legitimate allergy to a plaything. Pets may be the most perplexing case in point. Even without a formal program of pet therapy, children viewed their pets as sources of comfort, to hug and cuddle closely when sick. A pet could be an imagined protector or "guard dog," carrying a sense of security. A cooperative gerbil, rabbit, dog, or cat might be an ever-available play companion with whom to act out issues of illness. This was high irony if an allergy to the pet was at issue.

Seven-year-old Sean and his eleven-year-old brother both suffered from asthma. Their mother had asthma as a child and had empathy and compassion for the boys' misery. The day I met him, Sean confessed that animal hair, including that of rabbits, gerbils, guinea pigs, cats, and dogs, triggered his allergies. "First I get really itchy on my tear duct," he began. "Then little tears start coming … and then my face turns a little pink." Asthma symptoms could follow. Yet his mammal pets gave Sean great emotional comfort.

When Sean was discussing his fears of asthma, he suggested we should go see his hamster, Miss Storm, almost as if this would be a calming interlude. "She's not that much furry," Sean said to justify the risk, adding that the hamster did bite if handled the wrong way. Sean felt a connection to Miss Storm, as if his wishes mattered to the animal. "If I tell her to stop [running], she'll slow down a bit." The hamster had protective powers beyond its diminutive size. "If someone's really mad at me, and they try to beat me up, then she'll look at them really mad, and she bites when she's mad, so I'd put her on that person and she'd start going crazy getting him." Sean also had a bunny, purchased at a farm six weeks earlier with funds he and his teenage sister had saved. The bunny was kept in his sister's room. Sean handled the bunny but washed his hands carefully afterward. He admitted that he knew the bunny "would give him asthma." Washing hands, said Sean, "takes away the asthma because the asthma's on your hands." Another household pet was a snake belonging to Sean's eleven-year-old brother, a reptile that scared Sean even if it did not cause allergic symptoms. Sean and I laughed together about the irony of his being most scared of the animal that did not trigger asthma.

Despite the menagerie of pets in Sean's family, his mother, Mrs. Benson, did not approve of owning pets that made children sick. As a child, she explained, "my parents still had a dog, even though I suffered so." Yet she had agreed to have mammalian pets, since she knew how special pets could be, especially to a young animal lover like Sean. Sean had given up a dog, Petticoat, two years earlier. He had felt deeply attached to Petticoat and would lie on top of the dog in a full-body cuddle. Mrs. Benson understood that Sean would willingly trade discomfort for his pet, because he loved his dog so much. But Sean's need for medication started to increase after the family acquired Petticoat, and Mrs. Benson and his brother also needed increasing doses of their asthma medicines for relief.

Mrs. Benson found Petticoat a new family. This decision had been painful, of course. "I want Petticoat. I miss Petticoat. Can we get Petticoat back?" Sean had pleaded. But Mrs. Benson could not watch her children wheeze. She saw to it that her family could visit Petticoat at the dog's new home, which they still visited annually. Some visits had been tearful, since Petticoat clearly still recognized Sean and his family. In light of Sean's attachment to Petticoat, Mrs. Benson saw to it that Sean could send Petticoat a bone, pictures, and letters with the agreement of the new owners to share these mailings with Petticoat. One letter read, "I miss you Petticoat and I love you." The letters helped Sean cope with his grief; as Mrs. Benson speculated, "It was [Sean] showing Petticoat that he didn't forget about him." Mrs. Benson was willing to be sensitive to Sean's grief and took the trouble to provide avenues for Sean to express his feelings.

Sean grasped the issues involved when he discussed his former dog with me. "My dad didn't want us to take all the medicine, and we were suffering, and he didn't want us to suffer. So we had to give Petticoat away to these people that wanted a pet." Sean recalled with nostalgia how he had shared fun and confidences with his canine "best friend," yet the passing of time (and his mother's wise planning) had allowed him to better accept the loss of Petticoat. "That was past. Now I'm feeling better about it. Because my mom could have died, or we could have died, me or my brother."

Play with pets can help children cope with illness through companionship and pretense, even while ironically triggering symptoms. Play, whether with pets, people, or objects, entails a zone of trust that can be crucial to averting anxiety.[55] It is possible to manage necessary disruptions to the child's play, such as removing a pet, while leaving intact a child's general sense of safety and trust. Children seem to best endure the loss of a pet, or even a well-loved toy, when provided with tools for managing their feelings. In the Benson family, Sean was able to communicate his bond of affection with Petticoat, and his deeply felt grief, through gifts, letters, and visits. The parents' courage to willingly witness their child's painful feelings made it possible for Sean to work through the difficult loss.

Role-Reversal Play

The playful reversal by which the child dispenses care to a pet, toy, or playmate was among the most common types of medical play among diabetic and asthmatic children. Perhaps this is to be expected. Other research shows that terminally ill children often engage in role-reversal play as a means to enhance the child's sense of control over traumatic, invasive, painful, or disfiguring procedures.[56] Diabetic children in this study zealously took on the pretend role of doctor, parent, or veterinarian, dispensing shots through a toy syringe. The recipient might be a human playmate, a sibling, myself (as interviewer-playmate), or very often a toy animal or doll. Pantomimed blood tests were also administered to toys. When an empty inhaler included among the interviewer's toys was available for play, asthmatic children took the initiative to administer a "dose" to a doll or toy.

Role-reversal play allows children to rework present experience. The dramatized patient enacted by the doll, animal, or playmate takes over the role usually occupied by the child, allowing for company in misery, if only in pretense. Additionally, role-reversal play enables the child to take a controlling, rather than subordinate, fictive identity. The dialectic relationship of caregiver-receiver thus undergoes a dynamic reversal.

Sarbin, in discussing how adults appropriate characters when constructing identity, makes the case that identity is composite in nature.[57] That is, one's identity includes diverse role sets, although some aspects of identity may be pre-emptive and overriding. The sick role, as Parsons has described, carries with it deviant meanings that mesh poorly with a socially powerful identity.[58] Role reversal, on the other hand, sets forth a counter-signified role, symbolically weaving along with the sick role a more empowered strand of identity. Some children daydream about becoming physicians when they grow up, another strand of identity more powerful than the sick role.

The play by which ill children reverse roles and claim ascendancy over a play-patient implies a kind of fictive resistance by a usually subordinated child. Brian Sutton-Smith has asserted that children's play contains a "hidden rhetoric" about issues of power and identity.[59] Play helps children to vent and express their need to circumvent power by reversing positions.

This reversal of positions is a pattern also seen in other

contexts of human behavior. For example, many festivals incorporate a pattern whereby the lowly ascend and the mighty descend.
Halloween, in which children symbolically threaten to plunder
a treat from adults ("trick or treat"), has the markings of such a
reversal. So does the Bantu ritual in which one day is set apart
when usually subordinate women dress like men and do the jobs
of men.[60] In festival, role reversal serves a social function of re-
integrating social relations once the ritual is done. That is, the
usual subordination of children to adults or of Bantu women to
men is strengthened through the temporary inversion, through
upside-down balancing. In a clinical context, family therapists
have exploited the dynamic potency of role reversal by prescrib-
ing that a family explicitly carry out reversal exercises, such as
having the mother ask the children for help, as a way to shore up
relationships.[61]

By inverting the roles in treatment, then, children give expression to inequities and, by so doing, reconsider their identity
and position in the social order. As Erikson observed, children
"hallucinate" through play the very mastery and power they lack
at a given point in time.[62] Although this ploy may be less necessary
as children grow older and more capable of self-care, dependency
and subordination in early life are equilibrated by the play. Role-
reversal play destroys the social order by inversion yet sustains
current and future social relatedness in doing so. If play is a way
of vandalizing everyday social reality (as the patient "becomes" a
doctor), it also supports convention through rebalancing. Paradoxically, when a child takes free rein to playfully impersonate a
medical caretaker, this act shores up the child's acceptance of the
more subordinate role, patient. This is akin to what Bakhtin calls
"carnival ambivalence," in which festive participants overthrow
caste or rank, all with a strong element of play, in order to renew
their ongoing social relatedness.[63]

A well-worn truth among developmental psychologists recognizes that children engage in pretend play as an interim means to master significant material. The Swiss cognitive psychologist Jean Piaget appreciated this fact when one of his daughters, impressed by a dead duck lying on the kitchen table, the next day pretended to be a dead duck lying on the floor.[64] Piaget's Russian contemporary, Lev Vygotsky, also acknowledged the significance of pretend play during which a child uses the dialogue of imagined social action as a prior step toward internalizing social constructs. For Vygotsky, imagined conversation has transformative value by converting social interchange into inner recognition, all the while retaining the social nature of the learning.[65]

In role-reversal play, children imitate the discourse and behavior of caretakers. In turn, play provides an interim means for the child to understand the caretaker-patient relationship; this is, of course, a relationship fraught with social inequities and implied vulnerabilities. Role reversal equips the child to give substance to, and to transcend, the ambivalence. Note, then, that turnabout through "playing doctor" seems not to lead a child to rebel, but rather to better accept treatment. A child's playful opportunity to usurp the caretaker role shores up the child's consent to be a care-receiving patient.

Ritual

Play and ritual are related human processes. Both involve symbols to represent and act out events. Both involve a capacity to make-believe, in the sense of giving credence to, rather than critically analyzing, events. Both involve ambiguity of meaning, with room for contradictions, subversions, and absurdities or illogicalities. Finally, ritual and play both evade pat, logical reduction. Like play, ritual is recognizable and can have a discernible structure, yet the structure may disappear if one attempts to analyze and delineate the ritual beyond its encircling context. One point of difference between play and ritual is that ritual places more emphasis than play on regularity, precedent, and order. Ritual can contain not only the mysterious, but also the familiar, the element that is repeated every time. Indeed, one way to conceptualize ritual is to consider it as a mix of order with spontaneity, through a particular arrangement of symbols and actions.

Blood tests and insulin injections involve the regularity and familiarity of ritual, if only in the steps required to administer them. As mentioned earlier, diabetic children many times reserve a particular site on their body where they prefer to have (or not have) injections or other procedures. This, of course, exemplifies a goal of ordered familiarity.

Eight-year-old Janet Moore had never allowed her thumbs to be "poked" in four years of blood checks. She also considered her smallest fingers to be "safety fingers," drafted into service only if blood did not flow from the other fingers. Mrs. Moore thought that Janet's reserved fingers and thumbs represented a need for control and self-protection. Mrs. Moore therefore honored Janet's wishes about where to draw blood. With each blood test, Janet and her mother observed a shared ritual involving which body sites could not be touched, a way of evoking protection within a self-puncturing act.

Families practiced myriad rituals involving blood tests. A finger might be pressed until the bleeding stopped or might be dressed in a colorful plastic bandage. One child liked to be "pinched first" to establish a contrast with the level of pain from the puncture. One family used only colored lancets, inviting the child to choose which color would be used. Another family saved the tops that are removed from the lancets before each blood check and took a trip to a popular restaurant-arcade after accumulating a hundred tops; this provided a positive incentive and positive meaning for each test. One mother chose one week a year in which the child took a break from blood testing altogether. Some rituals involved the output, the numerical readings as to whether a child's blood sugar was high or low. If one boy had an overly high reading on a blood test, for instance, he could pronounce a preferred, fantasized rating number aloud, say, pronouncing that the number was an optimal 100, even though the actual number was double that. Another boy received a dollar if ever his numerical reading was 123 or 456.

Insulin injections included a variety of rituals, too, some of which have been described in other chapters. A telling example involved singing the refrain "Alleluia" from Handel's *Messiah,* a ritual practiced by a five-year-old boy, Tommy Dale In an interview Tommy's mother compared his "Alleluia" singing to the act of prayer, understandable to her as a distraction amidst the pain of injection. Her husband had suggested the practice to ameliorate the suffering during injections. "When I was a kid my sister told me at the dentist to pray to the Hail Mary." She laughed. "Kinda takes your mind off it. So Tom [Tommy's father] would say that to him about his shot. . . . I think my husband's nervousness about giving it to him is why . . . he wanted to settle him down."

The ritual suggested by Tommy's father was continued by his mother and further continued when the boy was in the care of a babysitter. From the mother's field notes:

FEBRUARY 4, 1996
Tommy says "Alleluia" several times while I give him his shot. His Dad tells him to say this, so he won't think about the shot.

FEBRUARY 5
He picks his leg for his shot this morning, again repeating "Alleluia" for the shot.

FEBRUARY 9
He said "Alleluia" for his shot in his leg.

From the babysitter's field notes:

FEBRUARY 11

He got a shot in his leg. He was singing 'Alleluia.' He was brave, didn't cry.

FEBRUARY 14

He got his shot, didn't cry, just sang "Alleluia."

And from the mother's notes:

FEBRUARY 25

Tonight Tommy had to write a song using A, C, and D for [music class]. He was determined and insistent he wanted to write "Alleluia" from Handel's Alleluia chorus. So we used different notes. . . . I wrote an explanation to the teacher [but] I did not explain why Alleluia (from when he gets his shots).

On the day of our final interview, Tommy had been singing Handel's rousing music throughout the day. It was evident that this melody was meaningful to him beyond mere distraction. The meaning of the activity seemed important to Tommy, since he sang "Alleluia" (and chose the song for a music class project) even apart from injections. The singing declared a victory of joy over adversity.

Distraction during childhood medical procedures has been demonstrated to ease distress during immunizations by watching cartoons;[66] to lower perceived pain during venipuncture by having a kaleidoscope to play with;[67] to decrease anxiety during genital examinations through the use of video eyeglasses;[68] to ameliorate pain and anxiety during IV insertion through distraction by a nurse;[69] and to lessen pain and distress during cancer-related procedures through film or story.[70] Studies have shown distraction to be a "well-established treatment" for procedure-related pain and distress.[71]

My home-based investigation of imaginal coping during procedures suggests that meaning, as well as distraction, is at work in the rituals. The meaning content of children's rituals is not random, not merely an arbitrary matter of drawing mental attention away from the pain. The ritual takes place in a social as well as a physical context and reflects emotional issues arising out of both the social and physical contexts. Ritual, like language or artistic expression, unfolds based on shared social momentum. The fact that children like to repeat the same ritualized actions across time supports the idea that particular coping rituals are personally satisfying at the level of meaning and feeling. Much like play, ritual reflects and sustains social reality, advancing human meaning, even without awareness. By setting out a framework of action, ritual can provide emotional support even when some participants have lost sight of needing support.[72] Ritual is thus powerful in its lasting impact, which holds up with habitual repetition, and indeed is enhanced by repetition.

When an asthmatic child asks her mother to clap to mark time when the child is using an inhaler, or cuddles under a special blanket during a nebulizer treatment, or keeps a favorite blue spacer nearby even after the doctor has switched prescriptions, this proclivity for ritual has a rationale, although it may not be a conscious one. Ritual evokes significance and can subtly draw out social recognition of meaning through its orderliness and drama. A child's needs are less dubitable, and potentially more collectively acknowledged, when they are given expression through ritual.

Within the family, ritual can clarify roles, thereby serving to establish and preserve a family's sense of itself, even under the pressures of a child's illness. Ritual is a bulwark of familiarity amidst the uncertainty of chronic illness. This enables the child to be more flexible in accepting difficult burdens. Ritual behavior serves the child and the child's family relationships amidst unrelenting, depleting obligations. Children bear unbearable affliction partly through the lift of ritual, sometimes hugging a teddy bear during treatment to do so.

Humor

Solomon, in Proverbs 17:22, states with solemn biblical authority that "a cheerful heart is a good medicine, but a downcast spirit dries up the bones." In modern times, medical research has accrued evidence that humor or laughter has palliative, healing impact. Experimental research with both adults and children points to the possibility that humor can reduce anxiety, moderate stress, or counter immunosuppression.[73] Experimental research is consistent with testimonial accounts, by patients reporting that humor is physically beneficial.[74]

Whether or not the wisdom of Solomon about humor is borne out by medical evidence, it is clear that humor has its place in the discourse of childhood illness. Laughter takes its cue from people interacting and draws on the common concerns of the joking participants.[75] In other words, shared laughter is based on a mutual definition of a situation. Given common meanings, humor connects those who are "in on" the joke, which is why comedy is useful to play therapists for building a bond with a child for clinical purposes.[76]

Humor also puts social meanings up for grabs, in that jokes mock and deride hard-and-fast categories of experience.[77] Humor is subversive, even as it constructs shared meaning, by introducing double meanings that freshly interpret what is ordinarily taken for granted. Humor can make a laughing stock of our habitual schemas and assumptions. For example, a joke can frame negative experience more positively or reframe serious suffering through irony.[78] Humor provides a kind of socially shared microvacation for the psyche by shifting us out of the usual taken-for-granted assumptions and offering another interpretation. In the process, comedy bends and derides normal frames of reference, even if only for a moment.

When humor touches children's understandings of their own illness experience, it can serve to reduce their stressful concerns. Consider, for example, an eight-year-old facing open-heart surgery who, by appreciating a joke, made light of his exposed predicament: "Eight-year-old Mark . . . was hospitalized for open heart surgery. [His ambition for adulthood was to be] a fireman, to 'put out fires.' The nurse's response that firemen are called to act quickly so that 'he might get caught with his pants down' elicited two minutes of laughter in the child who was so fearful of surgery." [79]

In American culture, professional clowns have a standing tradition of visiting hospitalized children. A clown, of course, is particularly qualified to poke fun at doctors, routines, and treatments that are fearful to a child, since clowns are culturally expected to function as jesters—as mockers of conventional authority. Clowns play the fool (sometimes the knowing fool), authorizing them to mock or shift meaning. [80]

Among the study sample of children with chronic illness, humor emerged spontaneously as part of daily social interaction (even though there were no clowns or funny nurses to assist). Humor was prevalent among children attending camp as well, as mentioned earlier. Mothers reported humor at home in their field notes.

APRIL 30, 1995

When I was giving Ann her 5:30 shot she said she hates diabetes, she wants to be able to eat whatever she wants. I said to her you can eat whatever you want as long as we fit it into our meal plan. She said I want to eat ice cream whenever I want. I said if you do you'll be a fatsy. I said no one should do that, we should eat good foods. We joked around about eating and getting fat—tried to make a joke out of it so she would . . . not feel so bad.

An eight-year-old girl with diabetes showed how humor was precipitated when she told of having a traumatic "low": "I laid down and fell asleep because I was so low. And then my mom couldn't wake me up. And I'm like"—she sighed to imitate the sounds of exhaustion. "I had dark circles around my eyes and I was very pale. And [my mother] said, um, she gave me some Life Savers, and glucose tablets, and then I was fine for a couple of minutes. . . . My mom went to call the ambulance because I was really low, and then my dad was giving me red Life Savers and I was coughing, like spitting them up. And the [medical] guy with the walkie-talkie was coming along, and he said 'She's spitting up blood! She's spitting up blood!'" She laughed at the medic's mistaking red Life Savers in her saliva for blood. "He thought I was really spitting up blood!" She ended her story, still laughing heartily at the misperception.

In these two examples from children with diabetes, a counter-normative aspect of diabetes was transformed by comic treatment: a prohibition on ice cream, in the first example, and a traumatic "low" crisis, in the second. Joking about being a "fatsy" converted the lack of ice cream into a restriction that no longer applied only to girls with diabetes, but in fact was a dietary precaution that should be widely followed. In the "low" crisis, the mirth over the mistaken "blood" recast the insulin reaction and life-saving ambulance visit as dubious in its threat, with an accompanying sense of comic relief (over a less daunting form of Life Savers). In both episodes, humor served to normalize rather than stigmatize, alleviating the danger or deprivation that was disruptive of the children's ordinary experience.

According to a theory posed by British comedian and physician Jonathon Miller, humor involves a dialectic dance of contrasting or ambiguous meanings.

> In my view, the value of humor may lie in the fact that it involves the rehearsal of alternative categories and classifications of the world in which we find ourselves. . . . When we are in the domain of humorous discourse—i.e. those cognitive situations which actually bring about laughter—we almost always encounter rehearsals, playings with, and redesignings of the concepts by which we conduct ourselves during periods of seriousness. When we conduct our ordinary . . . affairs, we deal with things for the most part by rule of thumb; we mediate our relationships with one another through a series of categories and concepts which are sufficiently stable to enable us to go about our business fairly successfully. But if we were rigidly locked on to these categories and concepts, if we were inflexibly attached to them, we would not continue to be a success-ful . . . species. What we require, then, is some sort of sabbatical let-out . . . to enable us to put things up for grabs: to reconsider categories and concepts so that we can redesign our relationships to the physical world, to one another, and even to our own notion of what it is to have relationships. . . . What I am suggesting is that [the] joke rehearses what we customarily think of as hard and fast divisions, . . . rejuvenates our sense of what everyday categories are. . . . By having gone through the delightful experience of humor, we have prevented ourselves from becoming the slaves of the categories by which we live.[81]

Humor enables suffering to take on a new arrangement and tone, as if reset to music not in minor key, but in a more upbeat major key. This was literally true at overnight camp for children with diabetes. Campers sang songs that merrily lampooned troubles, such as blood tests: "Don't take a prick at my finger, my finger. / Don't take a prick at my finger, my finger. / My finger *hurts*" [screamed loudly]. Another song mocked insulin reactions: "What a reaction, what a reaction, doodle lee do. / Some folks shake, and some get clammy, doodle lee do." Another song campers sang, part of a decades-old camp tradition, set tongue-in-cheek lyrics to the cheerful melody of Stephen Foster's "Oh, Susannah": "Oh I went to diabetic camp, / With my needle and my syringe. / They made me prick my finger, / 'Til I thought I would cringe." The song's chorus made a positive pronouncement on the campers themselves: "We came to diabetes camp, / And learned that we're the *best!*"

Children struck by illness, whose emergent selves face social and physical experiences that are isolating and threatening, need mechanisms to "put things up for grabs," to reframe and rede-fine—if only for the viability of their developing selves. Humor—along with play, story, and ritual—negotiates and vents some of the tension brought on by dissonant interpretations of person-hood. Humor empowers children to deal with the paradox of being both vulnerable and courageous, both exceptional and ordi-nary, both young and burdened. At home, some children acted "goofy" or enjoyed humor when they felt affronted or at risk, such as when they were talking about restrictions or fears in their lives. Distress before or after a particular threatening incident could be fodder for humor. Humor ameliorated everyday tension over self-affronting treatment. During insulin injections, a father would tell jokes, or a brother might make funny faces, assisting in the hu-morous engagement.

By virtue of being able to shift meaning about the self, joking qualifies as a "selfway," a means toward self-construction or re-making.[82] Chronic illness, like any life-threatening illness, severs the "normal" status of one's self and lifeworld, thereby unmooring the identity of the sufferer. Humor provides a kind of veiled rebel-lion against threats to self, making of the involved abnormalities an equilibrating remedy. Humor opens the possibility to lightly comment on the perilous and for the willing mind to consider a new interpretation.

Because laughter remakes meaning, it represents a dynamic of sanctuary from worry and constraint. "If you feel scared, and you start to laugh, do you remember that you're scared?" I asked a six-year-old boy with asthma. "No," he replied at once with a tone of sincerity. If, as in the popular song, whistling a happy tune can banish fear, so can humor allay threatening feelings. Children with a healthy funny bone considered the troubles they faced and refused to let despair take itself too seriously.

What Coping Entails

All the forms of imaginal coping introduced in this chapter involve ambiguity or a shift of meaning, such as that accomplished through story, ritual, play, or humor. Ambiguity allows for an active thought process that permits experience to be interpreted with license, perhaps with an accompanying emotional catharsis.[83] These imaginative discursive forms give voice to questions and doubts, and free us from becoming fixated on doubt. Ambiguity in a joke or ritual gives the coping process flexibility of meaning and thereby tensile strength. Humor, play, ritual, and story are interpretive potions of discourse, by which meaning is unconsciously, actively renegotiated.

Construing meaning amidst ambiguity is at once neither static nor predetermined, but rather is astir with nuance and flexibility. The ability to shift meaning (or "get" the joke) depends on the active participation of each interpreter, including, of course, the child. Humor, play, and ritual are pivot-points in meaning-making that hinge or turn upon the directional involvement of the child. In an experiment conducted among children on the first day of school, anxious students reduced their anxiety levels through using imagination in free play, better than a comparable group of anxious children who listened passively to a nature story.[84] Children who are coping through the use of fantasy are anything but passive. When a child uses cultural symbols borrowed from pop-culture superheroes or storybooks or toys, the child actively takes up the symbol and animates it for discourse. The resultant constellation of meaning, as Thomas Csordas suggests, is not attached to the symbol per se.[85] The meaning lies in the way the symbol is appropriated by the child, along with other social participants, who thereby redirect attention and remake significance. Symbols make shared actions and experiences meaningful, not in and of themselves, but largely through an active discursive process in which the child is central. The child's imagination constitutes a kind of "inner draftsman" who creatively crafts social and symbolic resources; this adept draftsman allows the child to animate her understandings and feelings about illness using complex, many-faceted symbolic material.[86]

Children have impressive capacities to interpret their social worlds, and they put these abilities to work in making and remaking sense of the thorny issues of illness. Experience, including past and present social interactions, influences this process. Scientific truths or medical authorities are not necessarily privileged over other sorts of messages or messengers. Nor does the child merely concentrate on negative outcomes and distress. Children, it seems, tap positive affect also as part of the alchemy of meaning, in the process infusing unhappy events with positive worth. This ability to reinterpret the unpleasant in a more positive light pervades how children use the tensile strength and flexibility of imaginal coping.[87]

This tensile strength, the capacity for adaptable meaning, is a prerequisite to coping with chronic illness. When illness interrupts the construed world of normal childhood, the child's selfhood no longer flows harmoniously amidst the norms in the world. The habitual hidden assumptions of social life break down. An aberration in the web of meaning, a violation of the child's world and identity calls for renegotiating the sense of things. It is as if the child needs to construct a renovated self and a refigured world from a fresh vantage point.[88]

Given that coping is inherently pivotal and transformative, it epitomizes a dynamic process. It is also a process that takes place in, and is affected by, a multifaceted social context. At illness camp or in families, individuals share dilemmas of meaning and rework meaning in concert. Meanings are derived from the tacit, interactive improvisation of the people involved and are not necessarily passively received from didactic indoctrination. Should a care provider wish to aid the child's coping, the first rule of business would be not to underestimate, undermine, dictate, or replace the child's own active, socially situated coping. Families in chronic illness face calamity in a manner more involved and impactful, and more meaning-based, than going through the surface motions of complying with a medical routine. Gaining the family's and child's cooperative involvement in treatment entails entering the family's and child's broader crisis of meaning. Care providers ignore the flexible lens of imagination at the peril of losing the strength and stretching needed to reframe illness in positive ways.

According to an African proverb, it is said that until lions have their historians, all tales of hunting will glorify the hunter. Very often, American tales of cure have glorified the physician or his allopathic allies. But it is the child, not the health care provider, who makes imaginal coping effective. On the level of meaning, the child is the principal healer and instigator of acceptance. The child is a key agent, when it comes to accepting treatment routines.

Given the importance of ongoing patient cooperation to the

treatment of chronic illness and the clinical outcome, caretakers cannot afford to ignore children's imaginations in the course of treatment. The poetic impulse of story, ritual, play, and humor can be powerfully therapeutic and empowering to the child— an advantage with potential for improving care, in ways not yet imagined.

CHAPTER 5

Children, Culture, and Coping

Our five and a half year old daughter has an inoperable brain tumor. Our only hope to remove the tumor is radiation. On the first day of her radiation treatment, she screamed and cried when she found out she would have to be in the room all by herself. . . . We kept saying that it would only take a minute. . . . Finally she asked me, "What is a minute?" . . . I looked at my watch and started singing, "It's a beautiful day in this neighborhood, a beautiful day for a neighbor," and before I could finish the song I said "Oops, the minute is up. I can't even finish Mr. Rogers' song." Then Michelle said, "Is that a minute? I can do that." And she did. She laid perfectly still for the entire treatment; but, there was a catch to it. I have to sing your song every time over the intercom.

LETTER TO FRED ROGERS

The soul would have no rainbow if the eyes had no tears.

NATIVE AMERICAN PROVERB

*T*his book offers a child-centered approach to understanding chronic illness. A child suffering from severe asthma or diabetes collides with a crisis of meaning, a kind of roadblock to significance within the child's lifeworld. Social dilemmas construct a block to meaning. The child's sense of self and world may be jolted when his personal eating practices clash with cultural practices at festive celebrations; a diabetic child cannot eat, for example, birthday cake or candy canes. Within cultural institutions like schools, a child comes face-to-face with her own exceptionality—as when asthma restricts her activities in gym class.

Viewing children's illness as a biomedical or physical event, without taking into account the broader expressive and social disruptions in children's lives, defeats understanding. Human beings, including children, interpret symbolic meaning and do so in a socially constituted world. The treatment for chronic illness presents both social and physical dilemmas to children. For example, chronically ill children are in some ways social outsiders, stigmatized by their illness and treatment. These children live in liminality, that is, a state of ambiguity, unsettledness, or confusion regarding the usual social categories.[1] Chronically ill children are unsettling to others, since they violate the cultural ideal of carefree, threat-free childhood. Treatment of their illness may involve taboo behaviors such as drawing blood or self-injection. Children with illness, even when they follow their treatment regimes to the letter, still suffer from being socially marginalized.

In coping with collisions of meaning, children use their facility at symbolic meaning-making, creatively manipulating symbols through play, ritual, story, humor, and even prayer. Vitality and adaptation are the hallmarks of coping among children, such as an eight-year-old boy who wrote the following prayers at school. (Prayer, of course is a form of imaginal coping, since it involves the use of the imagination in making contact with a transcendent, sacred realm.)

> Dear God,
> God you are cool. Can you find a cure for diabetes? It's kind of boring being a diabetic. Thank you for dying on the cross.
> Love, your pal, Todd.

A second letter was attached to a drawing of a tree, upon which, according to Todd, grew the cure for diabetes.

> Dear God,
> You're awesome. God, if you can find a cure for diabetes, thank you for everything you did for us. Love, Todd

Prayer points to hope in the midst of difficult experience through the envisioning of unseen possibilities. Prayer requires an act of faith, which necessitates some capacity to imagine the unseen, the transcendent. God is praised and asked for help, thanks to the scope of religious imagination.

Like children, adults also imaginatively reach out to cope amidst adversity, sometimes through prayer.[2] Psychologist Jacqueline Wooley and her colleagues have shown how adults think "magically" just as children do, citing data about adults who believe in ghosts, UFOs, and other occult phenomena.[3] Imaginal coping is not assumed to be a childhood artifact, but a mode of experience also found in adulthood. Indeed, adults from all societies call upon supernatural forces as a means of healing. Such practices as religious healing, shamanism, and mythic intervention are widespread across cultures, in some sense endorsing imaginal coping as a broad human phenomenon not limited to childhood.

James Dow, in an intriguing article on symbolic healing among adults, posits that symbolic healing by shamans, religious leaders, and so on follows a common pattern or structure. He found that healers, across societies, use culture-specific symbols and myths as media for healing. The healer persuades patients (or the patients persuade themselves) to view their personal problem in terms of the myth; the myth becomes a model or metaphor of the patient's experiences. The persuasion may involve trance, dreams, ecstatic experience, or other dramatizations that pose paradoxical frameworks. Once the mythic model is established, the symbols of the mythic frame are manipulated to suit a patient's dilemma in a way that couples the social context to the self of the patient, through symbols. In other words, the generalized symbols of myths are translated to the particular dilemmas of how patients see themselves in their social world. Emotions energize this process as much as cognition, according to Dow, including attention to one's own painful feelings, which signal the needed transformation.

Because culturally derived mythic worlds are vital repositories for symbols extracted for personal meaning, myths provide a "therapeutic lifeline to society."[4] Attacks on cultural myths will therefore be resisted. Whether through the patterned personal storytelling at Alcoholics Anonymous meetings or in a child's playful ritual, emotional transformation is tied to social values through symbolic structures.[5]

Dow acknowledges that cultural differences exist in the rate of resolution during healing, the content and structure of myths, and the assigned social role of the healer. In mainstream U.S. culture, my ethnographic study shows, children act as their own symbolic healers through imaginal coping. They adopt symbols from the cultural narratives of an age-graded society (Ninja Turtles, Power Rangers, Mister Rogers, etc.) and particularize these symbols to relate to personal dilemmas and feelings. While emotionally engaged with the myth, the symbols are manipulated in a healing transaction, such as imagining that the White Ranger has diabetes, or imagining that the Ninja Turtles will seek medical help in an emergency. Thus the cultural repertoire of stories and myths (as well as jokes, games, treatment rituals, and play routines) are a therapeutic lifeline for the child, helping to accommodate personal crises of meaning, of one's person or self within the social world.

This does not imply, however, that children's imaginal coping occurs through an identical process in all societies. Pretense in childhood takes a varied course in each social world. While Western middle-class adults may provide a supportive environment for pretend play, raising both the level and length of pretend-play episodes, pretense is not encouraged by adults in all societies. For instance, Mennonite or Amish children are discouraged from reading fairy tales or from engaging in pretend play (although they have access to religious myths). Less free time for pretending is available in Mennonite or Amish homes.[6] This cultural difference in childhood pretense likely creates important distinctions in how children use play to cope. Pretend play occurs infrequently in some non-Western societies, as well; the Mayans, for example, generally do not recognize play as a valuable activity for children.[7] Play (and imaginal coping) are activities best assessed within the cultural confines of the child's own lifeworld.

Individual differences may exist in each child's approach to play at particular times and in particular places. Some children intent on playing may do so even when they live in a society with minimal play resources. Historians document the remarkable ways in which children living in Nazi concentration camps used play during the Holocaust. With death all around them, children regarded death as a part of their world. One courtyard game consisted of children tickling a corpse. Children played in the yard outside the gas chamber, and at least one child danced in the waiting area just before death.[8]

Children do not choose the social world into which they are born, but they wondrously act to assimilate the realities of that world, no matter what the harrowing circumstances. Vitality and adaptation are hallmarks of young human beings.

It is the metaphoric structure of imaginal coping that is crucial to its shifts in meaning. Syringe-as-zebra, car-as-escape, wolf-as-asthmatic, or tiger-as-protector are a few examples of the ubiquitous use of metaphor among the children I studied. Anthropologist Gay Becker refers to metaphors as "mediators" in disrupted lives. By transposing meaning from one domain to another, metaphor names the nameless and accommodates coming to terms with the nameless. Metaphor enables bringing continuity amidst disruption, providing elasticity of meaning just when meaning needs reorganizing.[9]

During chronic illness, children use these metaphor structures and polyphonic meanings to reformulate their world. The impetus to do this is the unbearable nature of the illness experience.

As we have seen, children with asthma perceive on some level that life itself is at risk during breathing difficulty. Children with diabetes long for a cure, no matter how well they have adjusted to the daily routines of treatment and diet restrictions.

Treatment procedures for chronic illness are also enmeshed in the undoing of the child's lifeworld, as has been explained in earlier chapters. Despite the best medical intentions, prescribed interventions compromise meaning for the child and the family. Pain (from injections) may undo both parent (injector) and child (patient), as both feel their roles and identities subverted by the hurtful act. Families, the microsocieties of our culture, interact in mutual patterns of nurturance; this process is at risk when caring assumptions are undermined. Given that imaginal coping enhances the mutual roles of parent and child during hurtful procedures, this helps child and family alike.

Encumbered by profound difficulties, American children with a chronic illness work (or, better said, play and joke) to rebuild their realms of meaning. Imaginal coping carries heroic resilience. Still, chronic illness is no fairy tale, despite the imaginal coping of its young sufferers. Daily existence amidst treatment raises calls of distress, to which the power of imagination responds. This may not be a case of living happily ever after, but while a cure awaits, imagination mends.

Freeing Children's Voices

When talking to kids, you've got to pretend that you don't know much—and a few seconds later you realize you're not pretending.   BILL COSBY

In a poll conducted in May 1999, a cross-section of American children ages six to fourteen were asked, "What is bad about being a kid?" Perhaps to the surprise of some adults, children's answers didn't reflect unalloyed freedom and joy, even among healthy youngsters. At least some children felt "bossed around" (17 percent agreement); not able to do everything they wanted (11 percent); required to do schoolwork or homework (15 percent), to do chores (9 percent) or to be punished by "being grounded" (9 percent). Parents in the same survey mentioned only one of these misfortunes as a "bad" feature of childhood: homework (4 percent).[1] Adults easily miss the degree to which children's lives are encumbered by dependency and control.

It is frequently noted that institutionalized adult mental patients are "treated like children." The comparison is apt; both groups are subject to close monitoring, restriction of movement, and a lack of independent decision making.[2] The inference is that children are not treated the way adults ideally should be.

Child powerlessness is doubly the case for chronically ill children, who are dependent both by virtue of youth and by virtue of medical need. The uneven relationship between a chronically ill child and an adult caretaker or researcher can muffle the child's voice and perspective.[3] In a research setting, children are subordinate to the research process, such as with a test-like procedure administered by a directive adult.[4] The challenge in this inquiry was to inventively open the way to see the child's view—despite the imbalance that usually characterizes ill children's lives amidst adults.

In what follows, I will explain how I set about meeting the goal of freeing children's voices. Two approaches proved useful. First, I adopted an overall philosophy to pursue modes of study that were familiar and comfortable to children. Second, a tool kit of child-friendly methods (to be discussed shortly) served as a catalyst to children's comfort and communicating.

PREMISES OF THE STUDY

In undertaking this investigation, I recognized that childhood illness is an alloy of influences, including affect, cognition, body, culture, and especially the rich context of day-to-day existence. I wanted to do research that would allow me to hear about or witness (even indirectly) day-to-day life events for the child. Field notes kept by informant-mothers, and field notes kept at camp by researchers serving as camp counselors, provided a means for witnessing, indirectly, day-to-day events.[5]

The meanings held by children (and their parental caretakers) were central issues of interest. To explore issues of meaning, my interviews with children and parents were conducted twice in each family. These repeated interviews served to increase rapport over the course of our acquaintance. Children got to know me and, upon my return for the follow-up session, were excited to share with me their accomplishments, such as learning to give themselves injections or attending illness camp. Parents confided information in a follow-up interview that had not come out initially (such as confessing to cigarette smoking, despite having a child with asthma), as if barriers had been lowered with familiarity.

In making sense of interviews, field notes, and other material, I took an interpretive research approach. Interpretive research considers human action and culture to be ongoing processes of textlike construction.[6] That is, knowing, intending, deciding, desiring, and acting can be understood as "texts," as narrative or meaning-making processes mediated within symbolic communities. Interpretive research reflects the active role of human beings as they make inscriptions (rather than objective descriptions) of experience. Influential for these inscriptions are cultural, familial, and personal ways of rendering meaning.

From its inception, interpretive research has stirred questions. How are researchers to make sense of the human condition, if knowledge is symbolically mediated? If human experience is not charted objectively, how will researchers put things in any proper order? If humans do not have access to context-free truths, how can authoritative knowledge be possible?

Interpretive research invites looking at nuances of meaning, apart from authoritative knowledge. This might include confronting positions of privilege and indulging curiosity about those in overlooked social positions. To understand the illness experience, compassion for the young patient's own story bid me to rub out conventional lines of authority ordinarily marking what makes for valid knowledge. This heresy offered benefits, since it allowed a window into children's own worlds. I have tried to study illness squarely in the lifeworld of the child. I have aimed to produce what Van Manen calls "lived throughness," so that others might recognize experientially, through concrete examples, the resonance between the child's life and their own lived experience.[7] Wherever possible, I tried to foreground the children's roles in defining knowledge for themselves and framing their own experiences.

THE RESEARCH POPULATION AND SETTING

Let me start with the weather. The setting for this study was the Chicago metropolitan area, including urban and suburban areas. During the period of study (November 1992 through April 1996), Chicago had record-breaking heat spells as well as frigid subzero days. More than seven hundred died from heat in Chicago during the summer heat wave of 1995, during searing days when I darted in and out of an air-conditioned car to visit children's homes. Over the 1995 heat spell, the young asthmatic informants I visited stayed indoors to avoid the effects of the severe heat. Likewise, winter days of extreme cold made it dangerous for children with respiratory illness to be outside. The severe cold snap that took place during late January and early February 1996 (averaging nearly six degrees Fahrenheit) came close to breaking a ninety-seven-year record. Most children stayed in during that period, as well. The weather carried the inhospitable message of risk, especially for asthmatic children.

Among the forty-six families interviewed for this research, ten families were part of the pilot interview round, and thirty-six families were in the follow-up sample. Both samples were evenly split to include twenty-three children with diabetes and twenty-three children with asthma, overall. (This does not include siblings who also had diabetes, who were interviewed as well.) In the ten families from the pilot study, the children were ages seven through ten years, and included balanced numbers of both boys and girls. Based on pilot interviews that consisted of two home visits per family at intervals of about two months, it was decided that subsequent interviews should concentrate on very young children. Thus, the follow-up sample included thirty-six children ages five to eight, evenly split to represent diabetic and asthmatic children, with a balanced proportion of girls and boys.

Consistent with the pilot study, the follow-up investigation included two home visits per family, approximately two to three months apart. The home setting was chosen for two reasons. First, home is a "natural habitat" for children, a place where they are likely to feel secure and comfortable. Second, interviews at homes of children could shed new light on past research on childhood chronic illness, so often completed in hospitals or clinics (a common venue for clinical researchers).

In both waves of research, parental caretakers, usually mothers, kept field notes in the form of a notebook-diary during the time period between interviews. Since these records were kept by mothers intimately involved with the child emotionally and otherwise, it was not intended that these records would serve as objective, medical accounts of symptoms or treatment.[8] The field notes were meant to gain insights and observations about the children's daily lives, reported by adults close to them who observed and interpreted children's daily experience firsthand. Therefore, the parents were given a notebook with space on each page to fill in the date and instructed to "record your observations about your child's daily life with their illness and its treatment," but they were not trained to follow a particular structure or formal checklist of topics.

For the follow-up study, children were given a single-use camera and instructed to photograph "what it is like to have diabetes (or asthma)." Parental help with the photo-taking process was permitted and necessary, given the young age of the children. The pictures were developed before the second interview and served as a basis for the child to show and tell about their illness experience, using the photos.[9]

Collected research material was voluminous: interview transcripts, field notes, photos, and, in many cases, drawings done by children during interviews. A large file of recorded material accrued for each family I interviewed. Thousands of records in written and pictorial form comprised the basis for this book's interpretations.

Study participants (whose names are disguised in this book) were recruited by a professional research firm. A telephone questionnaire was administered to possible candidates for the study, to determine if the child and family qualified, that is, if the child met the study's definition for having diabetes or asthma. Based on initial interviews, children with asthma were screened in subsequent interviews using a delineated set of questions to parents, specifically prepared for this study, indicating severity and persistence of illness. Severe asthma was defined by asking the parent a three part question: Did the child use a peak flow meter? Did the child use prescribed medication continuously all year round? Did the child's medications include two or more different forms of medication, such as an oral form *and* an inhaler, or a nebulizer medication *and* another form? If parents responded affirmatively to at least two of these three questions, the child qualified, considered by the study to have severe asthma.

The investigation did not intend to make a comparative study of cultural subgroups, such as white suburban children versus inner-city children of color. Such cross-cultural comparisons, which are much needed, await future research.

THE ETHNOGRAPHER

Anthropologist Van der Geest has written that "the art of understanding is a melange of surprise and familiarity."[10] The surprise lies in the "otherness" of a way of life: Certain practices draw attention by contrasting with the usual practices of the examiner. At the same time, familiarity also coheres through a common ground between self and other, between informant and researcher. The paradoxical blend of strange with familiar enriches the research experience and is central to what is learned. As has long been said, the task of the ethnographer is to make the strange familiar, and to make the familiar strange. The encounter causes our own experience to be seen in fresh ways, even as it acquaints us more intimately with the experience of the other.

In studies of childhood chronic illness, the mix of surprise and familiarity has been characteristic. Approaching the study of illness is to meet the person (of any age) at a time of isolation, made more socially remote by stigma. The gap (a kind of exoticism) matters greatly, to the informant as much as the researcher. If the investigator shares any common ground with the ill party, a valued connection may be launched that reaches across the social distance usually engulfing illness.

I found that I could introduce myself to each child as both "other" and yet as one who has common ground. I have asthma that began at age nineteen, giving me at least some common ground with chronically ill children. With this knowledge, I introduced myself to each asthmatic child as someone who has asthma as an adult but did not have asthma as a child. I introduced myself to each diabetic child as having an illness (asthma), but not diabetes. I chose to reveal this information to each child as a disclosure of shared concern, yet an admission of ignorance and need to learn from the child. Although I was defined as a researcher ("a lady who likes to learn from kids"), I could traverse with the child both shared and distinctly "other" modes of understanding. Hortense Powdermaker wrote that an anthropologist is a "human instrument studying other human beings and societies," lacking ambitions to remove her personality from her work or to become a faceless recorder of events.[11] As an anthropological instrument, I wanted to connect with children as one human to another (and introduced myself as such), not to record impersonal, machinelike data with the indifference of detachment.

My willingness to be an open, empathic listener was an advantage as a researcher, although sometimes this was tenderly felt as a human being. I admit that I cried after some interviews over the suffering I'd just recorded and heard. Based on hearing so many children discuss the asthma experience, I became increasingly compassionate to the fine-tuned details of suffering from asthma, and thereby more aware of my own vulnerability. I began to feel my fragility in ways I had not before.

After my initial visit, children were eager for me to come again. Some waited outside, or next to the front window, for my arrival for the second interview. Two girls in different families dressed for the second interview by wrapping themselves in their special blankets (their transitional objects) before I arrived, inviting me to come to their room and "play some more," all the while engulfed in the safety of the blanket. The research seemed to be welcome therapy for many children, a chance to show and tell about ongoing stresses while snug in the comfort of home.

This work was challenging for me, but rewarding in the same measure as it demanded. It was a painstaking process to engage much younger "others" about their construal of illness. Like a play therapist, I had to bide my time and explore when each child seemed ready. There were awkward moments. One five-year-old boy spent an entire hour-long interview hitting me with his fist, while providing no verbal information about diabetes. Of course, this boy was actually telling me, in the best way he knew, his feelings of anger about a disease that would infuriate any of us. (His mother had another impression—that he was "used to it" by now, since he seemed on the surface to be cooperative with his treatments.)

In order to allow children to reveal their ideas at their own rate in a manner that felt safe, I used specially designed protocols of questioning that incorporated props and play. One method mentioned earlier used photo taking, and the photos served as a stimulus for the child's narration. This and other methods of interviewing will be described in the next section.

INTERVIEW TOOLS

As much as possible, I made each interview into a session of play, into which talk was inserted as relevant and natural to the play. I brought along a supply of toys, for instance, and generally shared these with the children as a way to learn about their asthma or diabetes. The toys included a cloth doll, which looked like Burt, the character from *Sesame Street;* a cloth doll resembling a white-faced, blond-braided girl; a toy doctor's kit, which opened to reveal a toy stethoscope; a toy thermometer; a toy syringe; a non-functional meter for testing blood glucose levels, if the child had diabetes; if the child had asthma, an empty inhaler, a spacer, a mask for a nebulizer, and a peak-flow meter; and a set of miniature hospital" props, complete with hospital bed, rolling hospital tray, an IV stand, figures of medical personnel, a toy blanket, and a miniature teddy bear.Children were invited to use the toy doctor's kit and dolls to show and explain "what happens" with their illness. Children had access to the hospital toys to narrate events when they visited or stayed in the hospital. If the child wanted, I would willingly play along with them, as a way of sustaining and focusing the discourse.

I also brought a tape recorder to use in recording our interactions. I invited each child to stop the tape recorder during our conversations, so that they could hear themselves—a diversion that was enjoyable for them.

The play during the interview was pleasurable to the children, who sometimes combined their personal toys with mine in their play. Play allowed children to present their side of the story in a way that came easily to them. Just as would be the case in play therapy, I treated the children as equals during this play, listened to them attentively, and treated their opinions with respect. I was rewarded with play sequences that implicitly explored the children's worlds and experiences.

> CDC: [Talks in the role of Burt doll] I'm gonna get sick and then what's gonna happen to me?
> BOY (age five): Everybody's gonna pinch your nose.
> CDC: [Asks Burt] Do people pinch your nose when you're sick? How come?
> BOY: [As Burt] Cause everybody hates me when I'm sick.
> CDC: Do you think she [referring to female doll] hates Burt when he's sick?
> BOY: No.
> CDC: What does she [the female doll] do for Burt?

BOY: Go get medicine. [Boy finds medicine in toy kit]

CDC: Now what should Burt do?

BOY: He should take it. [Shows how Burt takes off the cap of the inhaler, takes a big breath, and squirts]

CDC: After the medicine, does Burt feel like someone is holding his nose?

BOY: No.

CDC: He was feeling like somebody hated him. Does he feel that after?

BOY: No . . . he feels fine.

CDC: If he feels fine, what does he do?

BOY: Says thank you.

CDC: Who does he thank?

BOY: Her [refers to female doll] for getting the medicine.

In addition, I brought markers and paper to each interview. If a child was fond of drawing, I would incorporate picture making into the interview, inviting the child to draw. I would suggest as a drawing subject the worst time they ever remembered with their illness; or I'd ask for a drawing of what they imagined would happen on the day after their illness was cured. Some children produced numerous pictures. For children inclined toward art, the drawing was done with gusto and glee, as this mother's field notes convey.

DECEMBER 2, 1992

Today we were interviewed for a . . . study. After Taylor talked with Cindy about diabetes, he was very upbeat and animated. He said that he really enjoyed drawing pictures of his experience, hospital stays, shots, etc. It never occurred to me to do that with him. Next time, when he gets angry or upset about his disease, maybe we'll give him crayons and markers.

Other methods were specifically devised to explore children's feelings about the illness and its treatment. The most useful of these methods came to be known as the Metaphor Sort Technique

(MST).[12] The MST used the device of a picture sort; children looked through pictures and sorted them into two boxes, based on whether the picture had a feeling similar to that of the illness or treatment device. This sorting allowed children to communicate nonverbally and to express feelings. During the sorting process, children often gestured meaningfully with the picture—moved the picture to make the airplane fly, made a threatening gesture with the spider, and so on.

In one exercise from the MST, children were asked to sort through twenty-five pictures of places, ranging from a dark cave to a sunny playground to a burnt-down forest, and place them into one of two boxes. The children were asked to place pictures of places that had the same mood or feeling as their illness in a box known as the "asthma" or "diabetes" box. Conversely, pictures with a mood or feeling differing from the disease were to be placed in a separate box. The same depicted places were sorted regardless of whether a child was diabetic or asthmatic, though the disease in question was of course the child's own condition. This served as a nonverbal way for children to tell about the affective experience of their illness. They remained involved and communicative throughout the sorting task. Children conveyed a clear sense that the MST was well understood and provided a valuable way to communicate.

CDC: This is what we're gonna do. I'm gonna take your picture [drawing of child showing diabetes treatment] and put it underneath this [box], because that'll help us to remember that this is the diabetes box, and this is the not-diabetes box. [Points to each box] When you look at the picture [I show you now] a feeling is going to come to you, . . . and if that feeling is kind of like the way you feel about diabetes, it's gonna be attracted to this [diabetes] box like a magnet. Because this box has a strong diabetes feeling, right? But if it doesn't, it's gonna go "Uh oh" and go into this [non-diabetes] box. All right. [Holds out pictures, fanned face down, like a magician's cards]

Pick a card, any card. . . . As soon as you look at it, does it attract to the diabetes feeling? Or does it go in the other box?

GIRL: [Picks card of old house on hill, in a storm] This one, definitely . . . because diabetes makes me feel, like, kinda gloomy.

CDC: Uh huh. And this picture is kinda gloomy, and how else does it kinda feel?

GIRL: Creepy.

CDC: Creepy? Like what? Like what might happen?

GIRL: Cause it's like a haunted house, and it just has— [Makes a creepy face].

CDC: So there's a feeling to diabetes that something creepy could happen.

GIRL: Yeah, yeah.

CDC: What do you think that is?

GIRL: Like something could go wrong with you, and you'll have to go in the hospital and stay in the hospital much longer.

GIRL: [Chooses next picture] Sharks! [Backs off, dropping the card and then backing away] Creepy, creepy, creepy. [Places picture of sharks in diabetes box, under other pictures]

CDC: I think we'd better put these on the bottom. Too creepy! [Girl continues to choose and sort pictures]

In another MST variation, children were asked to sort through depictions of familiar objects shown in picture cutouts. The items to be sorted were chosen through pilot interviewing to include familiar objects that would encourage a range of responses. The sorted cutout pictures included a jack-in-the-box, a witch, a hand-held remote control, boxing gloves, a spider, a treasure chest, bubbles, lightning, a magic wand, a blanket, an ice skate, an airplane, a school bus, birthday cake candles, a bumblebee, a train, a batting helmet, a rainbow, a life jacket, red shoes (worn by Dorothy in the *Wizard of Oz*), a toothbrush, a car, a magic carpet, a teddy bear, an umbrella, a kite, a butterfly, a Christmas stocking, and a bomb. The instruction with these object-pictures was for the child to put objects that had the same mood or feeling as a particular treatment (such as injections) in one box, and objects with a different mood from their treatment in the other box. If children had more than one salient treatment (as most did), they were prompted to sort the set of objects repeatedly, for each salient treatment. Children viewed this visual sorting of object-pictures as a game and became involved in expressing how they felt about their treatments, through the visual metaphor.

> CDC: [As girl holds picture of baseball helmet above her head] The helmet's on your head, it feels like your nebulizer, how come?
> GIRL: The nebulizer is so boring, and a helmet is not very exciting.
> CDC: Okay [points to helmet], boring, boring, boring.
> GIRL: [Shows picture] An umbrella.
> CDC: What does an umbrella do?
> GIRL: So you won't get wet.
> CDC: Does a nebulizer do anything like that?
> GIRL: Yeah. It gives you air so you won't die.

The Metaphor Sort Technique enabled the child to express concerns, based on how the child sorted and interpreted each picture. Interpretations were at times particular to each youngster. One child chose the birthday cake, referring to its burning candles as hurtful, like an injection. Another child chose the birthday cake as a metaphor for injections but interpreted the cake as an emblem of good times, surrounded by friends.

Thanks to the MST, I did not need to directly ask about upsetting issues such as pain and anxiety but could listen for the child to raise such concerns through the chosen picture. This served as a protection for these young informants, since the children maintained control of whether and when to mention vulnerable topics. Even if a child had limited language skills, the metaphor provided a means to articulate feelings through image and gesture. The MST proved to be a very child-centered method that allowed young children to express abstract feelings through concrete, familiar objects. The process was gamelike to children, providing them with a welcome context to discuss their illness experience.

One drawback of the MST was that the objects sorted took on meanings that could fluctuate in the social context. A cartoon-style bomb (a sphere with a fuse) was originally included in the object sort, but I removed it when the Oklahoma City bombing occurred, in order not to frighten children. Pictures may reflect meanings of the real world, and these meanings may shift with world events.

Another method, chosen like the MST because it empowered children to tell their own story, made use of photographs. The photos were taken by the child and mother at my request using a single-use camera which I provided. The photos were then used as aids for describing the child's illness experience during a subsequent interview. (Two copies of each photo were made, so that the family could have a personal set of photos to keep.) This approach is referred to as an "autodrive" interview, since the informant selects and takes the photos and uses these to "drive" the interview.[13] Photo-assisted interviewing was a means to break through the power asymmetry in research, to authorize the child to both select and frame the issues. Children told their own stories at their own pace, at a rate and depth of disclosure they controlled. Discussion topics touched on fright, pain, anger, or other wounds, as these topics were initiated by the child, not by me.

Through the photo-assisted "autodrive" approach, children were able to peruse photos which they had a hand in making and to narrate their story, aided by the photographs.[14] Photos of treatment (injections and blood tests among diabetic children, or nebulizer treatments or medicine taking by asthmatic children) provoked explanations and associated feelings ranging from comfort and trust to irritation and pain. Children photographed instances of self-reassurance: sleeping with a special stuffed animal, bringing a trusted toy to the doctor's office, playing a ritual-like game along with their treatment, wearing a charm on their medical identification bracelet, and so on. Other photos gave rise to discussions of threatening situations: teasing by peers, at least one of whom could be seen flinching while watching a child's blood test; worry about death, especially during breath-depleting asthma episodes; or the ways in which adults underestimated their plight, such as in not realizing their degree of suffering, especially in asthma.

The autodrive approach both affected the process of the interview and guided its content, through photos. First, looking at the pictures with the child constituted a shared activity that readily established an egalitarian context. Merely by turning over or holding a photo, I could invite the child to give free recall about an event in a context distanced from immediate experience. This empowered the child to reflect on even traumatic experience in an "as if" manner, detached from the immediate circumstances. Events inciting anger or intense fear could be discussed in a reflective way, without any disruption of rapport. Children developed a striking degree of involvement, as the photos invited them to get it off their chests by recalling unpleasant happenings in a safe context, suitably distanced from events.

Finally, the photos served as tangible props useful to make reference to feelings or events. Photos could be sorted by children in a gamelike activity to identify categories of experience (e.g., by sorting the photos into piles of "good times" versus "bad times"). Another activity made use of plain white "thought balloons," the shapes that normally contain text in a comic strip, representing the thoughts of a character. By placing a thought balloon over the image of a child in a photograph, I could ask the interviewee to tell about an interior experience (private thought) through play with the thought-balloon sticker. The child remained highly involved during the task, while I gained a deeper understanding.

Children's framings of reality constitute singular social worlds which are pervasive, full of impact, and woefully underexplored. This study has identified some valuable ways to circumnavigate children's worlds from a youthful angle.

The reward has been a chance for children to revisit their lives and to meaningfully interpret events. For an adult respectful of children's modes of telling, these methods opened a way to penetrate children's otherness, and thereby become connected with their profound human plight.

A Primer for Adults

Sweet are the uses of adversity.

SHAKESPEARE, *AS YOU LIKE IT*

There are countless adults who are sensitive to children's needs for coping, including imaginal coping. Parents, often part of rituals during treatment, demonstrate how to be attentive and responsive to children's ways. Child-life specialists use play and other forms of imaginal coping to ease the experience of hospitalized children.

All caretakers have the opportunity to relate to children by acknowledging children's own claims about their lifeworlds. Some brief guidelines for doing so, which emerge as practical implications from this research, follow. These guidelines are based on research conducted at a particular time and place. Nevertheless, for the sake of adult practitioners who find the guidelines meaningful, I trace some general implications.

1. Do not assume that a child can be spared pain or suffering by avoiding discussion of difficult issues. Issues causing adult discomfort (such as the child's breathlessness, mortality, or pain) may well be crucial and salient to the child. Giving youngsters an opportunity to express their concerns will help to maintain common ground with them.

2. Do not assume that medical knowledge is a commodity to be taught didactically to the all-receptive child. Communication, since it is interactive, needs to allow for a child's ways of knowing, recognizing the active interpretation by the child. In other words, talk to children in their own language, in their own genre. Story, ritual, play, art, and humor hold active appeal for children. These

are poetic, metaphor-rich forms of discourse, able to communicate paradox and ambiguity, inviting children to interpret and reframe their experience. Expressive forms such as story (perhaps about a dying spider, or a wolf with asthma) help to build a community of meaning, as co-listeners improvise their personal, and at the same time shared or overlapping, meanings.[1] Story can build communities of support.

To communicate with children, take account of how they perceive, react to, and construe meaning within a particular domain. Design any communications to children (books, media, or personal presentations) in a manner which stays as close as possible to children's perceptions and unified experiences. A video, for example, that uses a teeter-totter to explain the balance between food, exercise, and insulin in diabetes hits a responsive chord with children's expertise about play, employing as a teaching vehicle a metaphor they seem to understand. Start with children's own knowing and check to be sure you are effectively communicating, if you intend to inform them.

3. Strive actively to understand the child's experience. The treatment regimen, as well as symptoms, may be central to the child's suffering. This means that the child may see as threatening what the adult sees as healing, even a seemingly innocuous peak-flow meter or newly prescribed inhaler. The child's construal of things will be essential in how the child accepts treatment. Children can dictate a failure of treatment, simply by their unwillingness to cooperate.

For children with diabetes and asthma, here are some additional guidelines:

1. Hospital treatment upon diagnosis of diabetes has a social impact at a symbolic or expressive level. A family checks into the hospital as a family that includes a child with diabetes, newly diag-

nosed. The same family checks out of the hospital as a family united and empowered, ready to confront diabetes. That is, hospitalization may serve as a "rite of passage" for the child and family, by which families obtain and co-construct a new identity and set of expectations. Hospitalization is culturally construed as a serious event, and can offer a transitional space set apart from ordinary social environments. Freed up from previous ways of being, a family with a hospitalized child transforms to incorporate the diagnosis. Explicit training in the procedures needed at home gives parents a chance to enact a new parental self, one charged and able to care for a chronically ill child. Emerging from the hospital, family members are no longer what they were. The family is set on a course of adjustment. Hospitalization may have healing value beyond its medical value, then, in providing a context for reforming identity and for family transformation. (When there is no hospitalization upon diagnosis, as is typical in asthma, the role change of the parents may be less consolidated, with less commitment to or acceptance of the treatment regimen.)

2. Families of children with asthma may benefit from measures that encourage parental acceptance. The repeated terror of asthma attacks brings about for children, and in some cases for parents, post-traumatic reactions and, in turn, passivity. Families of children with severe asthma need programs that therapeutically address the issue of fear, while empowering parents and children to effectively respond. Parents who themselves have experienced asthma attacks understand the terror their children undergo. Parents who are innocent of any personal experience with asthma may also be innocent of their child's intense suffering and may need to be apprised of the wrenching emotions involved, in order to sensitively respond to their child's experience. Children dislike some treatment interventions. Children with diabetes especially dislike injections, even if adults assume that children have become habituated. Children with asthma find the nebulizer especially

tedious and boring. The peak-flow meter also frustrates some children with asthma, who cannot win or succeed by "blowing all the way to the top." Efforts to improve the child's experience in using the syringe, nebulizer, and peak-flow meter, through redesign or revised instructions, would ameliorate children's hardship and perhaps contribute to fuller acceptance of the regimen.

3. Experiences with chronically ill peers (such as those at camp) can be especially valuable to children with asthma and diabetes. When in the company of peers, ill children are able to face up to and reframe the meaning of the burdens they share. Playful interactions, in an environment where illness behaviors are normative, seem to lighten the meaning of necessary regimens and afflictions.

4. Take account of the expressive hardships of chronic illness: the holidays and birthdays that cannot be fully observed due to diabetic food restrictions; the distancing, mocking, or trivializing reactions of others; the need to give up treasured possessions such as pets or stuffed toys, in asthma; or restrictions to stay indoors instead of play outside, in asthma. These expressive costs tax the child dearly. Efforts by adults that help children to engage fully in their social world in as normal a manner as possible are invaluable, such as providing sugar-free holiday treats for diabetics.

5. Adults who are sensitive to issues of meaning can have a significant therapeutic impact. Treatments lose their onerous quality, for example, when administered playfully. Conversely, treatments become hurtful when family-based rituals familiar to the child are unrecognized and unwittingly denied. Families' ritual practices such as play during treatment, or the use of comforting objects, should be tolerated, advocated, and appreciated as assets for coping.

Supporting imaginal coping entails an interactive role by the caretaker. When discussing which healing ritual should be chosen for psychotherapy, Hubble, Duncan, and Miller have remarked that the therapist should believe in the ritual and should show interest in the ritual.[2] No doubt, healing practices—play included—gain significance when rendered meaningful by the parent or care provider, as well as the patient. Imaginal coping is an opportunity for shared activity, for common ground between adult and child. Imaginal coping avoids an imposition of adult needs or desires upon the child quite apart from the child's own inclination. To be instructed in the corrective spells cast upon illness by imagination is to learn the child's own ways of playful relatedness and responsiveness.

Through the shared discourse of imaginal coping, treatments that could be onerous and isolating instead become rich with the bonds of shared meaning. There is no doubt that play can serve serious goals. The softest of toys can breach the harshest barrier of fear.

Notes

ACKNOWLEDGMENTS

1. Jane Wagner, *Search for Signs of Intelligent Life in the Universe* (New York: Harper and Row, 1986).

1: INTRODUCTION

1. Historically, when rates of childhood death were much higher, early death was less taboo. This is discussed in E. Hopkins, *Childhood Transformed: Working Class Children in Nineteenth Century England* (Manchester, Eng.: Manchester University Press, 1994), and Winterthur Museum, *Kids! Exhibit on Historic American Childhood* (Winterthur Museum: Winterthur, Del., 1999).

2. Dorothy Judd, *Give Sorrow Words: Working With a Dying Child* (New York: Haworth Press, 1995).

3. Asthma afflicts more than 4.4 million children under eighteen, comprising the most common chronic illness of youth in America. Moreover, asthma is spreading in its impact, with a 55 percent increase among children between 1982 and 1996. See American Lung Association, "Asthma in Children Fact Sheet," *http://www.lungsusa.org* (2002).

4. Christine Eiser, *Chronic Childhood Disease: An Introduction to Psychological Theory and Research* (Cambridge: Cambridge University Press, 1990); William Garrison and Susan McQuistin, *Chronic Illness During Childhood and Adolescence* (Newbury Park, Calif.: Sage, 1989); J. Hobbs, J. Perrin, and H. Ireys, *Chronically Ill Children and Their Families* (San Francisco: Jossey-Bass, 1985); M. Grey, M. Genel, and W. Tamborlane, "Psychosocial Adjustment of Latency-aged Diabetics: Determinants and Relationship to Control," *Pediatrics* 65 (1980): 69–73.

5. Between 1979 and 1989, the death rate for asthmatic children ages ten to fourteen rose 100 percent. National Center for Health Statistics,

National Health Survey, 1962–1990; American Lung Association, "Asthma in Children".

6. Methodological details, including the definitional criteria for recruitment of children with "severe asthma," are covered in Appendix A. Appendix A also discusses methodological issues and innovations in this study of childhood chronic illness.

7. Excellent qualitative investigations carried out in hospitals include: Ann Beuf, *Biting Off the Bracelet* (Philadelphia: University of Pennsylvania Press, 1979); Myra Bluebond-Langner, *The Private Lives of Dying Children* (Princeton: Princeton University Press, 1978); and David Bearison, *They Never Want to Tell You* (Cambridge: Harvard University Press, 1991). Myra Bluebond-Langner, *In the Shadow of Illness: Parents and Siblings of the Chronically Ill Child* (Princeton: Princeton University Press, 1996), deals with the families of cystic fibrosis patients, studied both in a hospital clinic and at home.

8. Programs of hospital play therapy, labeled under the rubric "child life," are described in J. Chan, "Preparation for Procedures and Surgery Through Play," *Pediatrician* 9 (1980): 210–219; J. Wilson, "Play in the Hospital," in C. Brown and A. Gottfried, eds., *Play Interactions: The Role of Toys and Parental Involvement in Children's Development* (Skilman, N.J.: Johnson and Johnson. 1985); C. Larsen, "The Child Life Professions: Today and Tomorrow," in *Child Life: An Overview* (Washington, D.C.: Association for the Care of Children's Health, 1986); D. Hymovich and G. Hagopian, *Chronic Illness in Children and Adults: A Psychosocial Approach* (Philadelphia: Saunders, 1992); and Evelyn Oremland, *Protecting the Emotional Development of the Ill Child: The Essence of the Child Life Profession* (Madison, Conn.: Psychosocial Press, 2000). The locations of ongoing child life programs are given in Child Life Council, *Directory of Child Life Programs* (Rockville, Md.: Child Life Council, 1996).

9. Underuse of peak-flow meters is also known from clinical reports, such as M. S. Kibirige, "Children Also Misinterpret the Signs," *British Medical Journal* 307 (1993): 1210.

10. D. Eisenberg, R. Kessler, C. Foster, F. Norlock, D. Calkins, and T. Delbianco, "Unconventional Medicine in the United States," *New*

England Journal of Medicine 328 (1993): 246−252; Meredith McGuire, *Ritual Healing in Suburban America* (Rutgers, N.J.: Rutgers University Press, 1994); Bonnie O'Connor, *Healing Traditions: Alternative Medicine and the Health Professions* (Philadelphia: University of Pennsylvania Press, 1995); Randy Potts, "Spirituality and the Experience of Cancer in an African-American Community," *Journal of Psychosocial Oncology* 14 (1996): 1−19; and J. Astin, "Why Patients Use Alternative Medicine: Results of a National Study," *Journal of the American Medical Association* 279 (1998): 1548−1553.

11. Biomedically trained physicians have also expressed views regarding the limits of strictly defined biomedicine, in works by noted authors: Arthur Kleinman, *The Illness Narratives: Suffering, Healing, and the Human Condition* (New York: Basic Books, 1988) and *Patients and Healers in the Context of Culture* (Berkeley: University of California Press, 1980); Jay Katz, *The Silent World of Doctor and Patient* (New York: Free Press, 1984); Oliver Sacks, *A Leg to Stand On* (New York: Harper-Collins, 1984); Bernie Siegel, *How to Live Between Office Visits* (New York: HarperCollins, 1986) and *Love, Medicine, and Miracles* (New York: Harper and Row, 1993); Arthur Weil, *Health and Healing* (Boston: Houghton Mifflin, 1988); and Deepak Chopra, *Ageless Body, Timeless Mind* (New York: Harmony Books, 1993). The National Institutes of Health has hosted meetings on alternative medicine, thereby recognizing such issues as "mind-body interactions" and community-based treatments. See National Institutes of Health, *Alternative Medicine: Expanding Medical Horizons* (Washington, D.C.: U.S. Government Printing Office, 1992).

2: JUVENILE DIABETES

1. "U of C Teams Head National Diabetes Research Project," *University of Chicago Magazine* 92:2 (December 1999): 19.

2. American Diabetes Association, *Children With Diabetes* (Alexandria, Va.: American Diabetes Association, 1986).

3. See B. Olsen, A. Sjolie, P Hougaard, J. Johannesen, K. Borch-Johnsen, K. Marinelli, B. Thorsteinsson, S. Pramming, H. Mortensen, and the Danish Study Group of Diabetes in Childhood 2000, "A

Six-Year Nationwide Cohort Study of Glycaemic Control in Young People With Type 1 Diabetes: Risk Markers for the Development of Retinopathy, Nephropathy, and Neuropathy," *Journal of Diabetes and Its Complications* 14 (2000): 295–300; Allen Lee Drash and Nina Berlin, "Juvenile Diabetes," in Nina Berlin and James Perrin, eds., *Issues in the Care of Children With Chronic Illness: A Sourcebook on Problems, Services, and Policies* (San Francisco: Jossey-Bass, 1985).

4. Byron Good, *Medicine, Rationality, and Experience: An Anthropological Perspective* (Cambridge: Cambridge University Press, 1994).

5. See this principle discussed in: Anne Fadiman, *The Spirit Catches You and You Fall Down* (New York: Noonday Press, 1997); Arthur Kleinman, *The Illness Narratives: Suffering, Healing, and the Human Condition* (New York: Basic Books, 1988) and *Patients and Healers in the Context of Culture* (Berkeley: University of California Press, 1980).

6. Byron Good, *Medicine, Rationality, and Experience*, 53.

7. The use of paraphrased and assembled material as a rhetorical device has considerable precedent in anthropological writing, such as in the construction of a daily scene from the life of a Mayan child; see Suzanne Gaskins, "Children's Daily Lives in a Mayan Village: A Case Study of Culturally Constructed Roles and Activities," in Artin Goncu, ed., *Children's Engagement in the World: Sociocultural Perspectives* (Cambridge: Cambridge University Press, 1999). Of late, qualitative researchers inside and outside of anthropology have spawned a range of alternative forms of ethnographic writing, extending to varied forms of assembled discourse. Such writing strategies are in keeping with Stephen Tyler's conviction that rhetorical approaches should be evocative of human experience with its complexity of voices; see Tyler, "Post-Modern Ethnography: From Document of the Occult to Occult Document," in James Clifford and George Marcus, eds., *Writing Culture: The Poetics and Politics of Ethnography.* (Berkeley: University of California Press, 1986).

8. Joan Austin, "Assessment of Coping Mechanisms Used by Parents and Children With Chronic Illness," *American Journal of Maternal Child Nursing* 15 (1990): 98–102; Ellen Perrin and P. Susan Gerrity,

"Development of Children With a Chronic Illness," *Pediatric Clinics of North America* 31 (1984): 19–31; John Lavigne and Joan Faier-Routman, "Psychological Adjustment to Pediatric Physical Disorders: A Meta-Analytical Review," *Journal of Pediatric Psychology* 17 (1992): 133–157; David Cadman, Michael Boyle, Peter Szatmari, and David Offord, "Chronic Illness, Disability, and Mental and Social Well Being: Findings From the Ontario Child Health Study," *Pediatrics* 79 (1987): 805–813.

9. Suzanne Johnson, Adrian Tomer, Walter Cunningham, and John Henretta, "Adherence in Childhood Diabetes: Results of a Confirmatory Factor Analysis," *Health Psychology* 9 (1990): 493–501; Margaret Grey, Myron Genel, and William Tamborlane, "Psychosocial Adjustment of Latency-Aged Diabetics: Determinants and Relationship to Control," *Pediatrics* 65 (1980): 69–73; Geoff Gill, "Psychological Aspects of Diabetes," *British Journal of Hospital Medicine* 46 (1991): 301–305; Margaret Grey, Mary Cameron, and Frances Thurber, "Coping and Adaptation in Children With Diabetes," *Nursing Research* 40 (1991): 144–149; O. Ryden, L. Nevander, P. Johnson, L. Westbom, and S. Sjoblad, "Diabetic Children and Their Parents: Personality Correlates of Metabolic Control," *Acta Paediatrica Scandinavica* 79 (1990): 1204–1212.

10. Sally Jacoby and Elinor Ochs, "Co-Construction: An Introduction," *Research on Language and Social Interaction* 28 (1995): 171–184.

11. Jean Lave and Etienne Wenger, *Situated Learning: Legitimate Peripheral Participation* (Cambridge: Cambridge University Press, 1991).

12. Good, *Medicine, Rationality, and Experience.*

13. Kathryn Hunter, *Doctors' Stories: The Narrative Structure of Medical Knowledge* (Princeton: Princeton University Press, 1991).

14. On learning to take case histories, see M. A. Milligan and E. S. More, *The Empathic Practitioner* (Rutgers, N.J.: Rutgers University Press, 1994).

15. Arnold Van Gennep, *The Rites of Passage* (Chicago: University of Chicago Press, 1960).

16. Caregiving in diabetes signals a relationship of care, similar to

the way cooking and feeding convey social connectedness to healthy middle-school children. Both food and caregiving enmesh children in relationships of care, symbolizing modes of giving and receiving by parents. See E. B. Kaplan, "Food as a Metaphor for Care," *Journal of Contemporary Ethnography* 29 (2000): 474–509.

17. Such feelings are compatible with attachment theory; for a history and review of this theory, see Inge Bretherton, "The Origins of Attachment Theory: John Bowlby and Mary Ainsworth," in R. Parke, P. Ornstein, J. Rieser, and C. Zahn-Waxler, eds., *A Century of Developmental Psychology* (Washington, D.C.: American Psychological Association, 1994).

18. Kenneth Gorfinkle, *Soothing Your Child's Pain* (Chicago: Contemporary Books, 1997).

19. The benefits of parental presence during hospitalization are widely accepted, as discussed in a review of the Ronald McDonald House charity that provides nearby housing for families when children are hospitalized far from home. See C. Sanford, "Ronald McDonald House: The House That Love Built," *Pediatric Nursing* 19 (1993): 260–262.

20. For a demonstration of how food transfers meaning (the "you are what you eat" principle), see Carol Nemeroff and Paul Rozin, "'You Are What You Eat': Applying the Demand-Free 'Impressions' Technique to an Unacknowledged Belief," *Ethos* 17 (1989): 50–69; Paul Rozin, "The Importance of Social Factors in Understanding the Acquisition of Food Habits," in E. Capaldi and T. Powley, eds., *Taste, Experience, and Feeding: Development and Learning* (Washington, D.C.: American Psychological Association, 1990).

21. Melanie Wallendorf and Eric Arnould, "Consumption Rituals of Thanksgiving Day," *Journal of Consumer Research* 18 (1991):17–31.

22. Among middle-school children, food serves as a metaphor for relationships of giving and receiving with parents and social institutions, conveying care. See Kaplan, "Food as a Metaphor for Care."

23. A full discussion of "passing" is included in Erving Goffman, *Stigma* (New York: Touchstone Press, 1963).

24. The meaning structure of Halloween is further discussed in

Victor Turner, *The Ritual Process: Structure and Anti-structure* (Ithaca, N.Y.: Cornell University Press, 1969). See also Russell Belk, "Halloween: An Evolving American Consumption Ritual," *Advances in Consumer Research* 17 (1990): 508–517; Jack Santino, "Halloween in America: Contemporary Customs and Performances," *Western Folklore* 42 (1983): 1–20; Jack Santino, *Halloween and Other Festivals of Life and Death* (Knoxville: University of Tennessee Press, 1994).

25. Sylvia Grider, "Conservatism and Dynamism in the Contemporary Celebration of Halloween: Institutionalization, Commercialization, Gentrification," *Southern Folklore* 53 (1996): 3–15.

26. Marcia Ory and Janine Kronenfeld, "Living With Juvenile Diabetes Mellitus," *Pediatric Nursing* 6 (1980): 47–50.

27. Mary Douglas, *Purity and Danger: An Analysis of Concepts of Pollution and Taboo* (New York: Praeger, 1966).

28. Janine Roberts, "Setting the Frame: Definition, Functions, and Typology of Rituals," in E. Imber-Black, J. Roberts, and R. Whiting, eds., *Rituals in Families and Family Therapies* (New York: Norton, 1988).

29. Waksler has shown, with regard to childhood in general, that adults often choose the preferred method even for common medical procedures, depriving children of having their preferences acknowledged. Such issues as whether a bandage is taken off slowly or quickly, whether pills are taken whole or crushed, or whether prayer or biomedicine is chosen as a preferred treatment are adult decisions, made for and imposed on the child. See Frances Waksler, *The Little Trials of Childhood* (London: Falmer Press, 1999); also see N. Walker, C. Brooks, and L. Wrightsman, *Children's Rights in the United States: In Search of National Policy* (Thousand Oaks, Calif.: Sage, 1999).

30. L. Monsaco, G. Geffken, and J. Silverstein, "Accuracy of Injection Site Identification Among Children With Insulin Dependent Diabetes Mellitus: A Comparison of Traditional and New Visual Aids," *Clinical Pediatrics* 35 (1996): 191–197. See also L. Siminerio and J. Betschart, *Children With Diabetes* (Alexandria, Va.: American Diabetes Association, 1986).

31. Didactic materials for diabetic children often address the

medical need for rotating injection sites; see, for example, J. Griffin, *Randy Has Diabetes* (Apache Junction, Ariz.: Edward's Publications, 1980).

32. Gorfinkle, *Soothing Your Child's Pain*, 94–95.

33. Malidoma Patrice Somé, *Ritual: Power, Healing, and Community* (New York: Penguin Books, 1993).

34. Sjaak Van Der Geest and Susan Reynolds Whyte, "The Charm of Medicines: Metaphors and Metonyms," *Medical Anthropological Quarterly* 3 (1989): 345–367.

35. Alan Prout, "Actor-Network Theory, Technology, and Medical Sociology: An Illustrative Analysis of the Metered Dose Inhaler," *Sociology of Health and Illness* 18 (1996): 198–219.

36. W. Liess, T. Kapellen, J. Siebler, J. Deutscher, K. Raile, A. Dost, K. Meyer, and U. Nietzchumann, "Practical Aspects of Managing Preschool Children With Type 1 Diabetes," *Acta Paediatrica Supplement* 425 (1998): 67–71; Siminerio and Betschart, *Children With Diabetes*.

37. For a vivid account of an adult's fear-inducing symptoms when in insulin reaction, see L. Rooney, *Sweet Invisible Body: Reflections on a Life With Diabetes* (New York: Holt, 1999).

38. For this definition of trauma, see Cynthia Monahon, *Children and Trauma: A Parents Guide to Helping Children Heal* (New York: Lexington Books, 1993), 1.

3: ENDURING CHILDHOOD ASTHMA

1. Data are taken from the database of: National Center for Health Statistics, U.S. Department of Health and Human Services, Centers for Disease Control, 2001. These estimates are based on children under age eighteen.

2. M. Wetzman, S. Gortmaker, A. Sobol, and J. Perrin, "Recent Trends in the Prevalence and Severity of Childhood Asthma," *Journal of the American Medical Association* 268 (1992): 2673–2677.

3. Nancy Sander, *A Parent's Guide to Asthma* (New York: Plume Books, 1994), xv.

4. Thomas Plaut, *Children With Asthma: A Manual for Parents* (Amherst, Mass.: Pedipress, 1988), 1.

5. J. S. Halterman, C. A. Aligne, P. Auinger, J. T. McBride, and P. G. Szilagyi, "Inadequate Therapy for Asthma Among Children in the United States," *Pediatrics* 105 (2000): 272–276; E. McCormick, "On the Rise: Asthma Among Children," *Pharmacy Times* 56 (1990): 90–92; W. Taylor and P. Newacheck, "Impact of Childhood Asthma on Health," *Pediatrics* 90 (1992): 657–662.

6. Data are derived from the National Center for Health Statistics. Note that out of 10,000 children affected by asthma in the United States, one will die from the disease. Researchers have also reported increased mortality from asthma in England, Wales, Australia, Canada, the Netherlands, Sweden, France, West Germany, Israel, and the United States. See C. Meza and M. Gershwin, "Why Is Asthma Becoming More of a Problem?" *Current Opinion in Pulmonary Medicine* 3 (1997): 6–9.

7. Sander, *A Parent's Guide*, 22–23.

8. McCormick, "On the Rise," 94.

9. Neil Buchanan and Peter Cooper, *Childhood Asthma: What It Is and What You Can Do* (Berkeley, Calif.: Tricycle Press, 1991).

10. There is strong and consistent evidence linking environmental tobacco smoke and childhood asthma, as described in D. Wartenberg, R. Erhlich, and D. Lilienfeld, "Environmental Tobacco Smoke: Comparing Exposure Metrics Using Probability Plots," *Environmental Research* 64 (1994): 122–135; P. Gergen, J. Fowler, and K. Maurer, *The Burden of Environmental Tobacco Smoke on the Respiratory Health of Children Two Months Through Five Years of Age in the United States* (AHCPR Publications Clearinghouse, 1998, at *http://www.pediatrics .org*).

11. Buchanan and Cooper, *Childhood Asthma*, 22. Similar findings are reported in W. Morgan and F. Martinez, "Risk Factors for Developing Wheezing and Asthma in Childhood," *Pediatric Clinics of North America* 39 (1992): 1185–1203.

12. See Appendix A for a full description of the study design, including the definition for "severe asthma" employed in selecting the study sample.

13. To better portray the illness experience, this chapter, like

chapter 2, incorporates first-person commentaries like the preceding ones, mosaics of edited discourse drawn from recurrent themes across numerous families.

14. Marian Uhlman, "Local Asthma Care Ineffective, Study Finds," *Philadelphia Inquirer*, November 8, 1998.

15. G. Becker, S. Janson-Bjerklie, P. Benner, K. Slobin, and S. Ferketich, "The Dilemma of Seeking Urgent Care: Asthma Episodes and Emergency Service Use," *Social Science in Medicine* 37 (1993): 305–313.

16. Not improving a child's home environment, that is, not acting on medical recommendations to air condition, switch to gas heat, or otherwise modify the home, is common. It is estimated that eliminating risky residential exposures would positively affect two million cases of asthma among children and adolescents. See B. Lanphear, R. Kahn, O. Berger, P. Auinger, S. Bortnick, and R. Nahhas, "Contribution of Residential Exposures to Asthma in U.S. Children and Adolescents," *Pediatrics* 107 (2001): E98.

17. Sander, *A Parent's Guide*, 28.

18. For additional details on asthma morbidity and death, see D. Ward, "An International Comparison of Asthma Morbidity and Mortality in U.S. Soldiers, 1984 to 1988," *Chest* 101 (1992): 613–620; F. Malveaux, D. Houlihan, and E. Diamond, "Characteristics of Asthma Mortality and Morbidity in African Americans," *Journal of Asthma* 30 (1993): 431–437; H. Rea, M. Sears, R. Beaglehole, J. Fenwick, R. Jackson, A. Gillies, T. O'Donnell, P. Holst, and P. Rothwell, "Lessons from the National Asthma Mortality Study: Circumstances Surrounding Death," *New Zealand Medical Journal* 100 (1987): 10–13; B. Miller and R. Strunk, "Circumstances Surrounding the Deaths of Children Due to Asthma: A Case-Control Study," *American Journal of the Diseases of Children* 143 (1989): 1294–1299.

19. A. Prout, L. Hayes, and L. Gelder, *Medicines and the Maintenance of Ordinariness and the Household Management of Childhood Asthma* (Staffordshire, U.K.: EU–BIOMED Project, 1996). This study found in ethnographic work that the inhaler is a key device by which parents maintain "ordinariness." From a child's perspective, the fact

that inhalers give personal control to restore freeness of breathing was important.

20. Further learning based on participant observation at illness camps is included in chapter 4.

21. See J. Campbell, "Illness Is a Point of View: The Development of Children's Concepts of Illness," *Child Development* 46 (1975): 92–100; E. Perrin and P. Gerrity, "There's a Demon in Your Belly: Children's Understanding of Illness," *Pediatrics* 67 (1981): 608–619; E. Perrin, A. Sayer, and J. Willett, "Sticks and Stones May Break My Bones . . . Reasoning About Illness Causality and Body Functioning in Children Who Have a Chronic Illness," *Pediatrics* 88 (1991): 26–30.

22. See J. Korbin and P. Zahorik, "Childhood, Health, and Illness: Beliefs and Behaviors of Urban American Schoolchildren," *Medical Anthropology* 9 (1985): 337–353.

23. For further discussion of children's intuitive theories, see S. Carey and E. Spelke, *Domain-specific Knowledge and Conceptual Change* (New York: Cambridge University Press, 1994); H. Wellman and S. Gelman, "Cognitive Development: Foundational Theories of Core Domains," *Annual Review of Psychology* 43 (1992): 337–375; and F. Keil, "The Origins of an Autonomous Biology," in M. Gunnar and M. Maratsos, eds., *Modularity and Constraints in Language and Cognition* (Mahwah, N.J.: Lawrence Erlbaum, 1992).

24. See B. Miller and B. Wood, "Childhood Asthma in Interaction With Family, School, and Peer Systems," *Journal of Asthma* 28 (1991): 405–414.

25. Similarly, research has shown that children as young as seven without chronic illness treat as salient the treatments of medicine, including medications and their ameliorative role. See A. Almarsdottir and C. Zimmer, "Children's Knowledge About Medicines," *Childhood* 5 (1998): 265–281.

26. See Arthur Kleinman's now classic work *The Illness Narratives: Suffering, Healing, and the Human Condition* (New York: Basic Books, 1988), in which Kleinman makes a similar argument, for adult patients, regarding the need to honor a patient's own version of events.

27. One important implication of children's non-biomedical conceptions of illness involves the communication between health care practitioners and children. Judging from my fieldwork, much of current didactic education falls short, since it assumes biomedical modes of thought about disease that are not aligned with children's own experiences and frameworks.

28. Ironically, some past studies of stress in childhood asthma, using questionnaires or checklists to assess which stresses are most troublesome, have failed to include breathlessness itself on the checklist; see, for example, M. Walsh and N. Ryan-Wengner, "Sources of Stress in Children With Asthma," *Journal of School Health* 62 (1992): 459−463. Based on such surveys, the social impact of asthma, including poor athletic performance and isolation from peers, has been better documented as stressful than has the terror of inadequate breathing.

29. See M. Davis and D. Wallbridge, *Boundary and Space: An Introduction to the Work of D. W. Winnicott* (New York: Brunner/Mazel, 1981).

30. V. Divertie, "Strategies to Promote Medication Compliance in Children With Asthma," *MCN: The American Journal of Maternal Child Nursing* 27(2002): 10-8; D. Cockcroft and F. Hargreave, "Outpatient Management of Bronchial Asthma," *Medical Clinics of North America* 74 (1990): 802.

31. See Appendix A for a description of the MST (Metaphor Sort Technique), which invited children to sort pictures having the "same feeling as asthma."

32. Gay Becker, *Disrupted Lives: How People Create Meaning in a Chaotic World* (Berkeley: University of California Press, 1997).

33. See S. Van Der Geest, "Grasping the Child's Point of View? An Anthropological Reflection," in P. Bush, D. Trakas, E. Sanz, R. Wirsing, T. Vaskilampi, and A. Prout, eds., *Children, Medicines, and Culture* (Binghampton, N.Y.: Pharmaceutical Products Press/Haworth Press, 1996), 342.

34. A. Prout, "Actor-Network Theory, Technology, and Medical Sociology: An Illustrative Analysis of the Metered Dose Inhaler," *Sociology of Health and Illness* 18 (1996): 199−200.

35. Prout, Hayes, and Gelder, *Medicines and Maintenance of Ordinariness* (n.p.).

36. In Frances Hodgson Burnett's *The Secret Garden* (New York: HarperCollins, 1987), the young characters use a garden as a special place of retreat, causing the decrepit garden to rejuvenate as the children themselves grow and heal; the secret garden is thus a magical place as well as a site of healing.

37. Van Der Geest, "Grasping the Child's Point of View."

38. Hopelessness, pessimism, or panic about asthma, along with worry over possible death, are themes also found in earlier research. See H. Yoos and A. McMullen, "Illness Narrative of Children With Asthma," *Pediatric Nursing* 22 (1996): 285–290; N. Clark, D. Evans, B. Zimmerman, M. Levison, and R. Mellins, "Patient and Family Management of Asthma: Theory-based Techniques for the Clinician," *Journal of Asthma* 31 (1994): 427–435.

39. Lenore Terr, *Too Scared to Cry* (New York: Basic Books, 1990).

40. Post-traumatic amnesia occurs among both adult and child survivors of trauma; see J. Herman, *Trauma and Recovery* (New York: Basic Books, 1997), 45–46.

41. Terr, *Too Scared to Cry.*

42. Edgar A. Poe, "Loss of Breath: A Tale Neither in nor out of Blackwood," *Edgar Allan Poe: Complete Tales and Poems* (New York: Barnes and Noble, 1993).

43. T. Brookes, *Catching My Breath* (New York: Times Books, 1994), 7.

44. Past studies of children's stress from asthma based on prestructured questionnaires typically have left unaddressed the life-connected meaning of breathing as a potential source of stress, focusing instead on less passion-stirring issues such as peer belonging or sports participation (e.g., Walsh and Ryan-Wengner, "Sources of Stress").

45. Myra Bluebond-Langner, *The Private Lives of Dying Children* (Princeton: Princeton University Press, 1978).

46. C. Kampfner, "Post-traumatic Stress Reactions in Children of Imprisoned Mothers," in K. Gabel and D. Jonston, eds., *Children of Incarcerated Parents* (New York: Lexington Books, 1995).

47. L. DeSalvo, *Breathless* (Boston: Beacon Press, 1997), 25, 76.

48. Terr, *Too Scared to Cry;* K. Alexander, "What Stories Mean to Children: Low-Income Preschoolers' Emotional Attachments to Stories" (Ph.D. diss., University of Illinois at Champaign-Urbana, 1996).

49. Cindy Dell Clark and Peggy Miller, "Play," in *Encyclopedia of Mental Heath* (San Diego: Academic Press, 1998).

50. As recently as 1968, clinical accounts of children with asthma were apt to conclude that the child suffered from an underlying "neurotic conflict" that produced and perpetuated the illness; see L. Burton, *Vulnerable Children: Three Studies of Children in Conflict* (New York: Schocken Books, 1968). The cycle of attacks and reactions was traced to a cause *within* the young victim, rather than recognizing that a threat was posed *to* the child from environmental factors. A similar notion was expressed by some adults I encountered in fieldwork, who viewed the asthmatic child as wheezing due to nervousness or maladjustment. Asthma, to them, was not a problem in itself, but an indicator of the child's psychological problems.

51. See M. Rich and R. Chalfen, "Showing and Telling Asthma: Children Teaching Physicians With Visual Narratives," *Visual Sociology* 14 (1999): 67.

52. For an excellent discussion of how traumas such as earthquakes also lead to ongoing anxiety through the undoing of assumptions about one's vulnerability and safety, see R. Janoff-Bulman, *Shattered Assumptions: Towards a New Psychology of Trauma* (New York: Free Press, 1992).

53. G. Deskin and G. Steckler, *When Nothing Makes Sense: Disaster, Crisis, and Their Effects on Children* (Minneapolis: Fairview Press, 1996).

54. A. Azarian and V. Skriptchenko-Gregorian, "Children in Natural Disaster," *Trauma Response* 4 (1998): 20–23.

55. In an inner-city self-management program aimed at children ages six to twelve, one of the facets most valued by children was the opportunity to express feelings. See V. Taggart, A. Zuckerman, R. Sly, C. Steinmuller, G. Newman, R. O'Brien, S. Schneider, and J. Bellanti, "You Can Control Asthma: Evaluation of an Asthma Education Pro-

gram for Hospitalized Inner-City Children," *Patient Education and Counseling* 17 (1991): 35–47.

56. Deskin and Steckler, *When Nothing Makes Sense.*

57. Rich and Chalfen, "Showing and Telling Asthma," 63.

58. Accounts of clinical experience suggest that parents gain skill and confidence as they meet with other mothers and fathers of asthmatic children. See, for example, Plaut, *Children With Asthma.*

59. A review of asthma education concluded that existing programs neither caused cats and dogs to be removed from the allergic individual's home nor affected smoking behavior. Indeed, it was concluded that both current patient-education materials and pamphlets and patient teaching in the clinical encounter had little effect on behavior. S. Wilson and N. Starr-Schneidkraut, "State of the Art in Asthma Education: The U.S. Experience," *Chest* 106 (1994): 197S–205S.

60. Janoff-Bulman, *Shattered Assumptions.*

61. A. Weinstein, *Asthma: The Complete Guide to Self-management of Asthma and Allergies for Patients and Their Families* (New York: Fawcett-Crest, 1987).

62. See Plaut, *Children With Asthma,* for an example of a book aimed at empowering parents through information.

63. Wilson and Starr-Schneidkraut, "State of the Art."

64. Barbara Sourkes, *Armfuls of Time: The Psychological Experience of the Child With Life-Threatening Illness* (Pittsburgh: University of Pittsburgh Press, 1995).

4: IMAGINAL COPING

1. M. Taylor, *Imaginary Companions and the Children Who Create Them* (New York: Oxford University Press, 1999).

2. Cindy Dell Clark, *Flights of Fancy, Leaps of Faith: Children's Myths in Contemporary America* (Chicago: University of Chicago Press, 1995).

3. Exceptions to the general dearth of research on imaginal thought include J. Wooley, "Thinking About Fantasy: Are Children Fundamentally Different Thinkers and Believers From Adults?" *Child Development* 68 (1997): 208–216; J. Wooley, K. Phelps, D. Davis, and

D. Mandell, "Where Theories of Mind Meet Magic: The Development of Children's Beliefs About Wishing," *Child Development* 70 (1999): 571–587.

4. E. Oremland, *Protecting the Emotional Development of the Ill Child: The Essence of the Child Life Profession* (Madison, Conn.: Psychosocial Press, 2000).

5. Erving Goffman, *Stigma* (New York: Touchstone Press, 1963).

6. Rich and Chalfen similarly found social embarassment about asthma treatments in a study in which teens with asthma videotaped daily life; M. Rich and R. Chalfen, "Showing and Telling Asthma: Children Teaching Physicians With Visual Narratives," *Visual Sociology* 14 (1999): 51–71.

7. For a review of research about the role of family in adjustment to chronic illness, consult W. Garrison and S. McQuiston, *Chronic Illness During Childhood and Adolescence: Psychological Aspects* (Newbury Park, Calif.: Sage, 1989). For a discussion of how families of children with cystic fibrosis act to maintain "normalcy and control," see Myra Bluebond-Langner, *In the Shadow of Illness: Parents and Siblings of the Chronically Ill Child* (Princeton: Princeton University Press, 1996), 186.

8. I share the view of cultural psychologists that it is important to examine cultural practices used by and around the child, since these practices are integrated, socially situated actions invested with significance. Practices that make up coping are forms of cultural practices. See Peggy Miller and Jacqueline Goodnow, "Cultural Practices: Towards an Integration of Culture and Development," in J. Goodnow, P. Miller, and F. Kessel, eds., *Cultural Practices as Contexts for Development* (San Francisco: Jossey-Bass, 1995); Barbara Rogoff, *Apprenticeship in Thinking* (New York: Oxford University Press).

9. See Eiser's review of coping research as it relates to childhood chronic illness: C. Eiser, *Chronic Childhood Disease: An Introduction to Psychological Theory* (Cambridge: Cambridge University Press, 1990).

10. This account is also described in Lenore Terr, *Too Scared to Cry* (New York: Basic Books, 1990), 238.

11. Posttraumatic play differs from normal play in its repetitive,

lifeless quality and "generally lacks both pleasure and relief" (Cynthia Monahan, *Children and Trauma: A Parent's Guide to Helping Children Heal* [New York: Lexington Books, 1993], 34). The lack of light-heartedness in play is a telling indicator that suggests childhood psychological trauma.

12. Studies supporting the value of camp include C. Kelly, S. Shield, M. Gowen, N. Jaganjac, C. Anderson, and G. Strope, "Outcome Analysis of a Summer Asthma Camp," *Journal of Asthma* 35 (1998): 165–171; A. Misuraca, M. Di Gennaro, M. Lioniello, M. Duval, and G. Aloi, "Summer Camps for Diabetic Children: An Experience in Campaniam, Italy," *Diabetes Research and Clinical Practice* 32 (1996): 91–96; A. Punnett and S. Thurber, "Evaluation of Asthma Camp Experience for Children," *Journal of Asthma* 30 (1993): 195–198; S. Fitzpatrick, S. Coughlin, J. Chamberlin, and Pediatric Lung Committee of the American Lung Association, "A Novel Camp Intervention for Childhood Asthma Among Urban Blacks," *Journal of the National Medical Association* 84 (1992): 233–237; G. Mimura, "Summer Camp," *Diabetes Research and Clinical Practice* 24 (1994): S287–S290; L. Sorrells, W. Chung, and J. Schlumpberger, "The Impact of a Summer Camp Experience on Asthma Education and Morbidity in Children," *Journal of Family Practice* 41 (1995): 465–468; W. Silvers, M. Holbreich, S. Go, M. Morrison, W. Dennis, T. Marostica, and J. Buckley, "Champ Camp: The Colorado Children's Asthma Camp Experience," *Journal of Asthma* 29 (1992): 121–135.

13. Kelly et al., "Outcome Analysis."

14. Punnett and Thurber, "Evaluation of Asthma Camp," 198.

15. Jay Mechling, "Children's Folklore in Residential Institutions," in B. Sutton-Smith, J. Mechling, T. Johnson, and F. McMahon, eds., *Children's Folklore: A Sourcebook* (New York: Garland, 1995).

16. More detail on the camps, and the ages of the campers at each camp, is included in Appendix A.

17. Taking a different but related view, Lave and Wenger discuss learning in terms of an "apprenticeship" in which the novice enters a community of masters, so that the novice affects the community as well as learning from it. Jean Lave and Etienne Wenger, *Situated Learning:*

Legitimate Peripheral Participation (Cambridge: Cambridge University Press, 1991).

18. See M. Bluebond-Langner, D. Perkel, T. Goertzel, K. Nelson, and J. McGeary, "Children's Knowledge of Cancer and Its Treatment: Impact of an Oncology Camp Experience," *Journal of Pediatrics* 116 (1990): 207–213.

19. Gary Alan Fine, "Small Groups and Culture Creation: The Idioculture of Little League Baseball Teams." *American Sociological Review* 44 (1979):733–745.

20. L. S. Vygotsky, "Play and Its Role in the Mental Development of the Child," *Soviet Psychology* 5 (1967): 6–18.

21. Mechling, "Children's Folklore," 291.

22. T. J. Scheff, "The Distancing of Emotion in Ritual," *Current Anthropology* 18 (1977): 483–505; T. J. Scheff, *Catharsis in Healing, Ritual, and Drama* (Berkeley: University of California Press, 1979).

23. According to Sawyer, play constitutes a kind of extended improvisation; see Keith Sawyer, *Pretend Play as Improvisation* (Mahwah, N.J.: Lawrence Erlbaum, 1997).

24. Among significant scholarly works in the 1990s espousing active and creative roles for children in interpreting and constructing culture are Jean Briggs, *Inuit Morality Play* (New Haven: Yale University Press, 1998); William Corsaro, *The Sociology of Childhood* (Thousand Oaks, Calif.: Pine Forge Press, 1997); William Corsaro and Peggy J. Miller, *Interpretive Approaches to Children's Socialization* (San Francisco: Jossey-Bass, 1992); Brian Cox and Cynthia Lightfoot, eds., *Sociogenetic Perspectives on Internalization* (Mahwah, N.J.: Lawrence Erlbaum, 1997); Alison James and Alan Prout, eds., *Constructing and Reconstructing Childhood* (London: Falmer Press, 1997); Rogoff, *Apprenticeship in Thinking*.

25. See Bruno Bettelheim, *The Uses of Enchantment* (New York: Vintage Books, 1977).

26. A written version of the three pigs story for asthmatic children, A. Zevy's *Once Upon a Breath* (Downsview, Ont.: Tumbleweed Press, 1997), takes a more didactic tack than the campers' version; campers

made no mention of this version. The story, financed by an educational grant from Glaxo Welcome, features a wolf with asthma who plays a saxophone, uses his "puffer" to relieve symptoms, and takes issue when the three pigs bring allergy-causing cats to his nightclub.

27. R. Murphy, *The Body Silent* (New York: Norton, 1990), 230–231.

28. For example, see Arthur Kleinman, *The Illness Narratives: Suffering, Healing, and the Human Condition* (New York: Basic Books, 1988); Arthur Frank, *The Wounded Storyteller* (Chicago: University of Chicago Press, 1995); K. Charmaz, "From the 'Sick Role' to Stories of Self: Understanding the Self in Illness," in R. Contrada and R. Asthmore, eds., *Self, Social Identity, and Physical Health* (New York: Oxford University Press, 1999); S. Taylor, L. Aspenwall, T. Giulano, G. Dakoff, and K. Reardon, "Storytelling and Coping With Stressful Events," *Journal of Applied Social Psychology* 23 (1993): 703–733.

29. See P. Miller, "Narrative Practices: Their Role in Socialization and Self-Construction," in U. Neisser and R. Fivsuh, eds., *Cultural Practices as Contexts for Development* (San Francisco: Jossey-Bass, 1994); P. Miller, R. Potts, H. Fung, L. Hoogstra, and J. Mintz, "Troubles in the Garden and How They Get Resolved: A Young Child's Transformation of His Favorite Story," in C. Nelson, ed., *Memory and Affect in Development* (Hillsdale, N.J.: Lawrence Erlbaum, 1990); P. Miller, J. Mintz, L. Hoogstra, H. Fung, and R. Potts, "The Narrated Self: Young Children's Construction of Self in Relation to Others in Conversational Stories of Personal Experience," *Merrill-Palmer Quarterly* 38 (1992): 45–67; P. Miller, A. Wiley, H. Fung, and C. Liang, "Personal Storytelling as a Medium of Socialization in Chinese and American Families," *Child Development* 68 (1997): 557–568; S. Van Deusen, S. Goldin-Meadow, and P. Miller, "Enacting Stories, Seeing Worlds: Similarities and Differences in the Cross-Cultural Narrative Development of Linguistically Isolated Children," *Human Development* 44 (2001): 311–336; A. Wiley, A. Rose, L. Burger, and P. Miller, "Constructing Autonomous Selves Through Narrative Practices: A Comparative Study of Working-Class and Middle-Class Families," *Child Development* 69 (1998): 833–847.

30. L. Cohen, "Bibliotherapy: Using Literature to Help Children Deal With Difficult Problems," *Journal of Psychosocial Nursing and Mental Health Services* 25 (1987): 20–24.

31. Miller et al., "Troubles in the Garden."

32. Bluebond-Langner, *Private Lives*, 128–134.

33. Many clinicians maintain that adults with unresolved traumatic experience achieve greater wholeness from story sharing. By this account, trauma's disruptive power lies in concrete perceptual images that interrupt coherence through involuntary flashbacks. In therapy, the adult constructs narrative depictions of distinctive episodes, and patient and therapist arrange and reassemble, out of the traumatic images, an organized, ordered, coherent story. David Pillemer, *Momentous Events, Vivid Memories: How Unforgettable Moments Help Us Understand the Meaning of Our Lives* (Cambridge: Harvard University Press, 1998).

34. Relevant reviews of the applied tradition of bibliotherapy, the use of story for therapeutic purposes, are given in S. H. Sclabassi, "Literature as a Therapeutic Tool: A Review of the Literature on Bibliotherapy," *American Journal of Psychotherapy* 17 (1973): 70–77, and J. Pardeck and J. Pardeck, *Bibliotherapy: A Clinical Approach for Healing Children* (Yverdon, Switz.: Godron and Breach Science, 1993). The use of story to address stress from childhood illness is discussed in A. Fosson and E. Husband, "Bibliotherapy for Hospitalized Children," *Southern Medical Journal* 77 (1984): 342–346, and N. Parikh and M. Schneider, "Book Buddies: Bringing Stories to Hospitalized Children," *School Library Journal* 35 (1988): 35–39. Examples of bibliotherapy in other domains include C. Carlile, "Children of Divorce," *Childhood Education* 67 (1991): 232–234; G. Farkas and B. Yorker, "Case Studies of Bibliotherapy With Homeless Children," *Issues in Mental Health Nursing* 14 (1993): 337–347; A. Klingman, "Biblioguidance With Kindergartners: Evaluation of a Primary Prevention Program to Reduce Fear of the Dark," *Journal of Clinical Child Psychology* 17 (1988): 237–241; R. Lenkowsky, M. Dayboch, E. Barowsky, L. Puccio, and B. Lenkowsky, "Effects of Bibliotherapy on the Self-Concept of Learning Disabled, Emotionally Handicapped Adolescents in a

Classroom Setting," *Psychological Reports* 61 (1987): 483–488; J. Pardeck, "Children's Literature and Child Abuse," *Child Welfare* 69 (1990): 83–88; J. Pardeck and J. Pardeck, "Bibliotheraphy for Children in Foster Care and Adoption," *Child Welfare* 69 (1987): 269–278; M. E. Walker, "When Children Die: Death in Current Children's Literature and Its Use in a Library," *Bulletin of the Medical Library Association* 74 (1986):16; and T. Hebert, "Meeting the Affective Needs of Bright Boys Through Bibliotherapy," *Roeper Review* 13 (1991): 207–212.

35. See R. Riordan, "Bibliotherapy Revisited," *Psychological Reports* 68 (1991): 306.

36. K. J. Alexander, "What Stories Mean to Children: Low-Income Preschoolers' Emotional Attachments to Stories" (Ph.D. diss., University of Illinois, 1996).

37. Taylor, *Imaginary Companions;* D.W. Winnicott, "Transitional Objects and Transitional Phenomena," *Collected Papers* (New York: Basic Books, 1958).

38. Examples of toys that come alive in fictional treatment are discussed in L. Kuznets, *When Toys Come Alive: Narratives of Animation, Metamorphosis, and Development* (New Haven: Yale University Press, 1994).

39. Regarding the soothing value of imaginary companions, including in medical situations, see Taylor, *Imaginary Companions.*

40. For a discussion of imaginal relationships of adults, see Ted Sarbin, "The Poetics of Identity," *Theory and Psychology* 7 (1997): 67–82; J. Caughey, *Imaginary Social Worlds* (Lincoln: University of Nebraska Press, 1984).

41. See S. Fish, *Is There a Text in This Class? The Authority of Interpretive Communities* (Boston: Harvard University Press, 1980).

42. The videotape "It's Time to Learn About Diabetes" is available through Chronimed Publishing (800-848-2793). The use of a teeter-totter as a metaphor for diabetes was memorable to children from this teaching video, consistent with the documented educational value of metaphors in science education. See K. Tobin and D. Tibbins, "Metaphors as Seeds for Conceptual Change and the Improvement of Science Teaching," *Science Education* 80 (1996).

43. This suggestion—taking into account how children perceive, react, and construct meaning—also applies to the minimal effectiveness of current asthma education materials reported in S. Wilson and N. Starr-Schneidkraut, "State of the Art in Asthma Education: The U.S. Experience," *Chest* 106 (1994): 197S–205S.

44. E. Erikson, *Childhood and Society* (New York: Norton, 1950), 44, 45.

45. On the social significance of play, see the work of Lev Vygotsky, a major scholar of play in a social context, who echoed Erikson in his theories that play offers developmental advantages in the social context: L. Vygotksy, *Mind in Society* (Cambridge: Harvard University Press, 1978); *Thought and Language* (Cambridge: MIT Press, 1986); and "Play and Its Role."

46. On the cognitive importance of play, see J. Piaget, *Play, Dreams, and Imitation in Childhood* (New York: Norton, 1962).

47. On play's variation among cultures, see W. Haight, X. Wang, H. Fung, K. Williams, and J. Mintz, "Universal, Developmental, and Variable Aspects of Young Children's Play: A Cross-cultural Comparison of Pretending at Home," *Child Development* 70 (1999): 1477–1488; S. Carlson, M. Taylor, and G. Levin, "The Influence of Culture on Pretend Play: The Case of Mennonite Children," *Merrill-Palmer Quarterly* 44 (1998): 538–565; A. Goncu, J. Tuermer, J. Jyoti, and J. Johnson, "Children's Play as Cultural Activity," in A. Goncu, ed., *Children's Engagement in the World: Sociocultural Perspectives* (Cambridge: Cambridge University Press, 1999).

48. In one exceptional study, Zeltzer and Lebaron reviewed the use of fantasy in helping a child to cope in a therapeutic context, acknowledging that such coping may also occur spontaneously. These authors concluded that systematic study is needed of chronically ill children's spontaneous coping using fantasy. See L. Zeltzer and S. Lebaron, "Fantasy in Children and Adolescents With Chronic Illness," *Developmental and Behavioral Pediatrics* 7 (1986): 195–197.

49. This finding is consistent with a survey of coping strategies used by eight- to thirteen-year-olds attending asthma camp that found 48 percent self-reported "cuddling a pet or stuffed animal" when cop-

ing; N. Ryan-Wenger and M. Walsh, "Children's Perspectives on Coping With Asthma," *Pediatric Nursing* 20 (1994): 224–228.

50. Byron Good, *Medicine, Rationality, and Experience: An Anthropological Perspective* (Cambridge: Cambridge University Press, 1994); L. Hunt and C. Mattingly, "Diverse Rationalities and Multiple Realities in Illness and Healing," *Medical Anthropological Quarterly* 12 (1998): 267–272.

51. See R. Hausner, "Medication and Transitional Phenomena," *International Journal of Psychoanalytic Psychotherapy* 11 (1986): 375–398. Placebos place meaning and belief at the center of the therapeutic encounter, as positive belief confers on placebos their efficacy or acceptance. The role of belief is relatively disregarded in biomedicine. See D. Morris, "Placebo, Pain, and Belief: A Biocultural Model," in A. Harrington, ed., *The Placebo Effect: An Interdisciplinary Exploration* (Cambridge: Harvard University Press, 1997).

52. One study found that healthy children used a transitional object more when they experienced intense hassles, suggesting that Rick's use of a blanket in the face of worries may also occur with pressures other than illness; S. Lookabaugh and V. Fu, "Children's Use of Inanimate Transitional Objects in Coping With Hassles," *Journal of Genetic Psychology* 153 (1992): 37–45.

53. How the imagination lends itself to preparation for future role taking is discussed in S. Taylor, L. Pham, I. Rivkin, and D. Armor, "Harnessing the Imagination: Mental Simulation, Self-Regulation, and Coping," *American Psychologist* 53 (1998): 703–733.

54. I. D'Antonio, "Therapeutic Use of Play in Hospitals," *Nursing Clinics of North America* 19 (1984): 351–359.

55. Winnicott, "Transitional Objects."

56. Barbara Sourkes, *Armfuls of Time: The Pyschological Experience of the Child With Life-Threatening Illness* (Pittsburgh: University of Pittsburgh Press, 1995).

57. Sarbin, "The Poetics of Identity."

58. T. Parsons, *The Social System* (New York: Free Press, 1951).

59. Brian Sutton-Smith, *The Ambiguity of Play* (Cambridge: Harvard University Press, 1997).

60. E. Imber-Black, J. Roberts, and R. Whiting, eds., *Rituals in Families and Family Therapies* (New York: Norton, 1988), 318.

61. O. Van der Hart, *Rituals in Psychotherapy* (Boston: Houghton-Mifflin, 1988).

62. See Erikson, *Childhood.*

63. M. Bakhtin, "Carnival Ambivalence," in P. Morris, ed., *The Bakhtin Reader* (London: Arnold Press, 1994).

64. Related in A. Goncu and S. Gaskins, "The Role of Pretense and Language in the Development of Self," *Human Development* 41 (1998): 200–204.

65. Vygotsky, "Play and Its Role."

66. L. Cohen and G. Panopoulos, "Nurse Coaching and Cartoon Distraction: An Effective and Practical Intervention to Reduce Child, Parent, and Nurse Distress During Immunizations," *Journal of Pediatric Psychology* 22 (1997): 355–370.

67. J. A. Vessey, K. L. Carlson, and J. McGill, "Use of Distraction With Children During an Acute Pain Experience," *Nursing Research* 43 (1994): 369–372.

68. A. B. Berenson, C. M. Wiemann, and V. I. Rickert, "Use of Video Eyeglasses to Decrease Anxiety Among Children Undergoing Genital Examinations," *American Journal of Obstetrics and Gynecology* 178 (1998): 1341–1345.

69. D. Fanurik, J. L. Koh, and M. L. Schmitz, "Distraction Techniques Combined With EMLA: Effects of IV Insertion Pain and Distress in Children," *Children's Health Care* 29 (2000): 87–101.

70. C. Kleiber and D. Harper, "Effects of Distraction on Children's Pain and Distress During Medical Procedures: A Meta Analysis," *Nursing Research* 48 (1999): 44–49.

71. S. W. Powers, "Empirically Supported Treatments in Pediatric Psychology: Procedure-Related Pain," *Journal of Pediatric Psychology* 24 (1999): 131–145.

72. S. Wolin and L. Bennett, "Family Rituals," *Family Process* 23 (1984): 401–420.

73. For adults, see L. Berk and S. Tan, *Laughter and the Immune System: A Serious Approach* (Meadville, Pa.: Touchstar, 1996); N. Yo-

vetich, A. Dale, and M. Hudak, "Benefits of Humor in Reduction of Threat-Induced Anxiety," *Psychological Reports* 66 (1990): 51–58; R. Martin and J. Dobbin, "Sense of Humor, Hassles, and Immunoglobin A: Evidence for the Stress-Moderating Effect of Humor," *International Journal of Psychiatry in Medicine* 18 (1988): 93–105; A. M. Johnson, "A Study of Humor and the Right Hemisphere," *Perceptual and Motor Skills* 70 (1990): 995–1002; P. Wooten, *Compassionate Laughter: Jest for Your Health* (Salt Lake City: Commune-A-Kay, 1996). For children, see R. Lambert and N. Lambert, "The Effects of Humor on Secretory Immunoglobin A Levels in School-Aged Children," *Pediatric Nursing* 21 (1995): 16–19.

74. A notable example is Norman Cousins, *Anatomy of an Illness* (New York: Norton, 1979).

75. H. Bergson, *Laughter* (*Indypublish.com*, 2002).

76. J. LeVine, "The Clinical Use of Humor in Work With Children," in P. McGhee and A. Chapman, eds., *Children's Humor* (New York: Wiley, 1980).

77. Jonathon Miller, "Jokes and Joking: A Serious Laughing Matter," in J. Durant and J. Miller, eds., *Laughing Matters: A Serious Look at Humor* (Essex, U.K.: Longman, 1988).

78. K. Locke, "A Funny Thing Happened! The Management of Consumer Emotions in Service Encounters," *Organization Science* 7 (1996): 40–59; R. Coser, "Some Social Functions of Laughter: A Study of Humor in a Hospital Setting," *Human Relations* 12 (1959): 176.

79. Irma D'Antonio, "The Use of Humor With Children in Hospital Settings," in P. McGhee, ed., *Humor and Children's Development* (New York: Haworth Press, 1989), 167.

80. Linda Miller Van Berkon, "Clown Doctors: Shamanic Healers of Western Medicine," *Medical Anthropology Quarterly* 9 (1995): 462–475.

81. Miller, "Jokes and Joking," 11.

82. H. Markus, P. Mullaly, and S. Kitayama, "Selfways: Diversity in Modes of Cultural Participation," in U. Neisser and D. Jopling, eds., *The Conceptual Self in Context* (New York: Cambridge University Press, 1997).

83. Scheff, *Catharsis in Healing.*

84. L. Barnett, "Young Children's Resolution of Distress Through Play," *Journal of Child Psychology and Psychiatry* 25 (1984): 477–483.

85. T. Csordas, "The Rhetoric of Transformation in Ritual Healing," *Culture, Medicine, and Psychiatry* 7 (1983): 333–375.

86. The notion of the imagination as "inner draftsman" is borrowed from L. Goldman and C. Smith, "Imagining Identities: Mimetic Constructions in Huli Child Fantasy Play," *Journal of the Royal Anthropological Institute* 4 (1998): 207–234.

87. Coping influenced by positive affect is central to the argument of S. Folkman and J. Moskowitz, "Positive Affect and the Other Side of Coping," *American Psychologist* 55 (2000): 647–654.

88. See B. Babcock, "Arrange Me Into Disorder: Fragments and Reflections on Ritual Clowning," in J. MacAloon, ed., *Rite, Drama, Festival, Spectacle: Rehearsals Towards a Theory of Cultural Performance* (Philadelphia: Institute for the Study of Human Issues, 1984).

5: CHILDREN, CULTURE, AND COPING

1. J. Willett and M. Deegan, "Liminality and Disability: The Symbolic Rite of Passage of Individuals With Disabilities," paper presented at the American Sociological Association annual meeting, Washington, D.C., 2000.

2. L. Dossey, *Prayer Is Good Medicine* (New York: HarperCollins, 1996); Potts, "Spirituality and the Experience."

3. J. Wooley, K. Phelps, D. Davis, and D. Mandell, "Where Theories of Mind Meet Magic: The Development of Children's Beliefs About Wishing," *Child Development* 70 (1999): 571–587.

4. J. Dow, "Universal Aspects of Symbolic Healing: A Theoretical Synthesis," *American Anthropologist* 88 (1986): 56–69.

5. L. Goldman and C. Smith, "Imagining Identities: Mimetic Constructions in Huli Child Fantasy Play," *Journal of the Royal Anthropological Institute* 4 (1998): 207–234.

6. S. Carlson, M. Taylor, and G. Levin, "The Influence of Culture on Pretend Play: The Case of Mennonite Children," *Merrill-Palmer Quarterly* 44 (1998): 538–565.

7. Suzanne Gaskins, "How Mayan Parental Theories Come Into Play," in C. Super and S. Harkness, eds., *Parents' Cultural Belief Systems: Their Origins, Expressions, and Consequences* (New York: Guilford, 1996).

8. G. Eisen, *Children and Play in the Holocaust* (Amherst: University of Massachusetts Press, 1988), 105, 67.

9. Gay Becker, *Disrupted Lives: How People Create Meaning in a Chaotic World* (Berkeley: University of California Press, 1997).

APPENDIX A

1. C. Wallis, "The Kids Are Alright," *Time*, July 5, 1999, 56–58.

2. E. Goffman, *Asylums: Essays on the Social Situation of Mental Patients and Other Inmates* (Garden City, N.Y.: Anchor Books, 1961).

3. A discussion of the child's dependent role and the need for research that privileges children's viewpoints is given in J. Korbin and P. Zahorik, "Childhood, Health, and Illness: Beliefs and Behaviors of Urban American Schoolchildren," *Medical Anthropology* 9 (1985): 337–353.

4. The point that children can be disempowered by research is discussed in the context of institutionally based (such as school-derived) research in R. Edwards and P. Alldred, "Children and Young People's Views of Social Research: The Case of Research on Home-School Relations," *Childhood* 6 (1999): 261–281.

5. All three camps were studied during summer 1995. Camp 1 was a two-day camp held in daytime only. The children observed at this camp were six and seven years old and had diabetes. Their siblings were also invited to camp. Camp 2 was seven days long, an overnight camp for eight- to twelve-year-old children with diabetes. Camp 3 was a seven-day overnight camp for children with asthma. The counselors who served as participant-observers were chosen for their research aptitude and received training before the start of camp. One was a medical student, one worked in research, and one was a registered pharmacist and business student.

6. Cynthia Lightfoot, "The Clarity of Perspective: Adolescent Risk

Taking, Fantasy, and the Internalization of Cultural Identity," in B. Cox and C. Lightfoot, eds., *Sociogenetic Perspectives on Internalization* (Mahwah, N.J.: Lawrence Erlbaum, 1997).

7. M. Van Manen, "From Meaning to Method," *Qualitative Health Research* 7 (1997): 345–369.

8. Diary records of symptoms kept by adults have been shown to lack consistent accuracy and therefore are a questionable method of following symptoms. M. Hyland, C. Kenyon, R. Allen, and P. Howarth, "Diary Keeping in Asthma: Comparison of Written and Electronic Methods," *British Medical Journal* 306 (1993): 487–489.

9. This technique of the "autodriven interview" with children is discussed in Cindy Dell Clark, "The Autodriven Interview: A Viewfinder into Children's Experience," *Visual Sociology* 14 (1999): 39–50. The technique is derived from adult or adolescent interviewing techniques discussed by Deborah Heisley and Sid Levy, "Autodriving: A Photoelicitation Technique," *Journal of Consumer Research* 18 (1991): 252–272, and Lenore Butler, "Autodrive in Qualitative Research: Cracking the Ice With Young Respondents," *Canadian Journal of Market Research* 13 (1994): 71–74.

10. S. Van Der Geest, "Grasping the Children's Point of View? An Anthropological Reflection," in P. Bush, D. Trakas, E. Sanz, R. Wirsing, T. Vaskilampi, and A. Prout, eds., *Children, Medicines, and Culture* (Binghamton, N.Y.: Pharmaceutical Products Press/Haworth Press, 1996).

11. Hortense Powdermaker, *Stranger and Friend: The Way of an Anthropologist* (New York: Norton, 1966), 1.

12. Cindy Dell Clark, "Illness as Visual Metaphor: Visual Props in a Study of Childhood Chronic Illness," paper presented at the American Sociological Association annual conference, Washington, D.C., 2000.

13. Clark, "The Autodriven Interview"; Heisley and Levy, "Autodriving."

14. In a similar approach using videotape, patients ages eight to nineteen made videos of their asthma experiences to show to their physicians. M. Rich and R. Chalfen, "Showing and Telling Asthma:

Children Teaching Physicians With Visual Narratives," *Visual Sociology* 14 (1999): 51–71.

APPENDIX B

1. Jerome Bruner, *Acts of Meaning* (Cambridge: Harvard University Press, 1990), and *Actual Minds, Possible Worlds* (Cambridge: Harvard University Press, 1986).

2. See M. Hubble, B. Duncan, and S. Miller, *The Heart and Soul of Change* (Washington, D.C.: American Psychological Association, 1999).

Selected Bibliography

Ahluvalia, T., and Schaefer, C. 1994. "Implications of Transitional Object Use: A Review of Empirical Findings." *Psychology, a Journal of Human Behavior* 31(2):45–57.

Aldwin, C. 1994. *Stress, Coping and Development: An Integrative Perspective.* New York: Guilford Press.

Almarsdottir, A. and Zimmer, C. 1998. "Children's Knowledge about Medicines." *Childhood* 5(3):265–281.

American Diabetes Association. 1986. *Children with Diabetes.* American Diabetes Association.

American Lung Association. 1992. *Asthma: What Every Parent Should Know.* Rochester, NY: American Lung Association.

American Lung Association. 2002. "Asthma in Children Fact Sheet." *http://www.lungusa.org.*

Applegate, J. 1989. "The Transitional Object: Some Sociocultural Variations and Their Implications." *Child and Adolescent Social Work* 6(1):38–51.

Apte, M. 1985. *Humor and Laughter: An Anthropological Approach.* Ithaca: Cornell University Press.

Austin, J. 1990. "Assessment of Coping Mechanisms Used by Parents and Children with Chronic Illness." *American Journal of Maternal Child Nursing* 15:98–102.

Azarin, A. and Skriptchenko-Gregorian, V. 1998. "Children in Natural Disaster." *Trauma Response* 4:20–23.

Azarnoff, P. and Flegal, S. 1975. *A Pediatric Play Program.* Springfield, IL: Charles C. Thomas Publishers.

Azarnoff, P. and Lindquiest, P. 1997. *Psychological Abuse of Children in Health Care: The Issues.* Tarzana, CA: Pediatric Projects Inc.

Babcock, B. 1984. "Arrange Me Into Disorder: Fragments and Reflections On Ritual Clowning." In *Rite, Drama, Festival, Spectacle:*

Rehearsals Towards a Theory of Cultural Performance, edited by J. MacAloon. Philadelphia: Institute for the Study of Human Issues.

Bakhtin, M. 1994. "Carnival Ambivalence." In *The Bakhtin Reader,* edited by P. Morris. London: Arnold Press.

Barnett, L. 1984. "Young Children's Resolution of Distress through Play." *Journal of Child Psychology and Psychiatry* 25(3):477–483.

Bearison, D. 1991. *They Never Want to Tell You.* Cambridge, MA: Harvard University Press.

Becker, G. 1997. *Disrupted Lives: How People Create Meaning In A Chaotic World.* Berkeley: University of California Press.

Becker, G., Janson-Bjerklie, S., Benner, P., Slobin, K., and Ferketich, S. 1993. "The Dilemma of Seeking Urgent Care: Asthma Episodes and Emergency Service Use." *Social Science in Medicine* 37(3):305–313.

Beeman, W. 2000. "Humor," *Journal of Linguistic Anthropology* 9(2).

Behr, S. and Murphy, D. 1993. "Research Progress and Promise: The Role of Perceptions in Cognitive Adaptation to Disability." In *Cognitive Coping, Families, and Disability,* edited by J. Turnbull, S. Behr, D. Murphy, J. Marquis, and M. Blue-Banning. Baltimore: Brookes Publishing.

Berenson, A. B., Wiemann, C. M., and Rickert, V.I. 1998. "Use of Video Eyeglasses to Decrease Anxiety among Children Undergoing Genital Examinations." *American Journal of Obstetrics and Gynecology* 178(6):1341–1345.

Bergson, H. 1980. *Laughter.* Baltimore: Johns Hopkins Paperback.

Berk, L. and. Tann, S. 1996. *Laughter and the Immune System: A Serious Approach.* Meadville, PA: Touchstar.

Bettelheim, B. 1977. *The Uses of Enchantment.* New York: Vintage Books.

Beuf, A. 1979. *Biting off the Bracelet: A Study of Children in Hospitals.* Philadelphia: University of Pennsylvania Press.

Bluebond-Langner, M. 1978. *The Private Worlds of Dying Children.* Princeton: Princeton University Press.

Bluebond-Langner, M. 1996. *In the Shadow of Illness: Parents and Siblings of the Chronically Ill Child.* Princeton: Princeton University Press.

Bluebond-Langner, M., Perkel, D., and Goertzel, T. 1991. "Pediatric cancer patients' peer relationships: The impact of an oncology camp experience." *Journal of Psychosocial Oncology* 9:67–80.

Bluebond-Langner, M., Perkel, D., Goertzel, T., Nelson, K., and McGeary, J. 1990. "Children's Knowledge of Cancer and Its Treatment: Impact of an Oncology Camp Experience." *The Journal of Pediatrics* 116(2):207–213.

Briggs, J. 1998. *Inuit Morality Play.* New Haven: Yale University Press.

Brody, S. 1980. "Transitional Objects: Idealization of a Phenomenon." *Psychoanalytic Quarterly* 49.

Brown, J. 1993. "Coping with Stress: The Beneficial Role of Positive Illusions." In *Cognitive Coping, Families and Disability,* edited by A. Turnbull, J. Patterson, S. Behr, D. Murphy, J. Marquis, M. Blue-Banning. Baltimore: Paul H. Brookes Publishing.

Buchanan, N. and Cooper, P. 1991. *Childhood Asthma: What It Is and What You Can Do.* Berkeley: Tricycle Press.

Busch, F. 1974. "Dimensions of the First Transitional Object." *The Psychoanalytic Study of the Child* 29:215–228.

Busch, F. 1977. "Theme and Variation in the Development of the First Transitional Object." *International Journal of Psychoanalysis* 58:479–486.

Cadman, D., Boyle, M., Szatmari, P., and Offord, D. 1987. "Chronic Illness, Disability, and Mental and Social Well Being: Findings from the Ontario Child Health Study." *Pediatrics* 79: 805–813.

Campbell, J. 1973. "Illness Is A Point of View: The Development of Children's Concepts of Illness." *Child Development* 46:92–100.

Carlson, S., Taylor, M., and Levin, G. 1998. "The Influence of Culture on Pretend Play: The Case of Mennonite Children." *Merrill-Palmer Quarterly* 44(4):538–565.

Cassell, S. 1965. "Effect of Brief Puppet Therapy upon the Emotional Responses of Children Undergoing Cardiac Catheterization." *Journal of Consulting Psychology* 29(1):1–8.

Caughey, J. 1984. *Imaginary Social Worlds.* Lincoln, Nebraska: University of Nebraska Press.

Chafe, W. 1987. "Humor as a Disabling Mechanism." *American Behavior Scientist* 30(1):16–26.

Chan, J. 1980. "Preparation for Procedures and Surgery through Play." *Pediatrician* 9:210–219.

Chapman, A. and Foot, H. 1976. *Humor and Laughter: Theory, Research and Applications.* London: John Wiley and Sons.

Charmaz, K. 1999. "From the 'Sick Role' to Stories of Self: Understanding the Self in Illness." In *Self, Social Identity and Physical Health,* edited by R. Contrada, and R. Asthmore. New York: Oxford University Press.

Christiano, B. and Russ, S. 1996. "Play as a Predictor of Coping and Distress in Children during an Invasive Procedure." *Journal of Clinical Child Psychology* 25:130–138.

Clark, C. D. 1996. "Interviewing Children in Qualitative Research: A Show and Tell." *Canadian Journal of Marketing Research* 15:74–79.

Clark, C. D. 1998. "Childhood Imagination in the Face of Chronic Illness." In *Believed-in Imaginings: The Narrative Construction of Reality,* edited by J. DeRivera and T. Sarbin. Washington, DC: American Psychological Association.

Clark, C. D. 1999a. "The Autodriven Interview: A Photographic Viewfinder into Children's Experience." *Visual Sociology* 14:39–50.

Clark, C. D. 1995. *Flights of Fancy, Leaps of Faith: Children's Myths in Contemporary America.* Chicago: University of Chicago Press.

Clark, C. D. and Miller, P. J. 1998. "Play." *Encyclopedia of Mental Health.* San Diego: Academic Press.

Clark, N., Evans, D., Zimmerman, B., Levison, M., and Mellins, R. 1994. "Patient and Family Management of Asthma: Theory-Based Techniques for the Clinician." *Journal of Asthma* 31(6):427–435.

Cockcroft, D. and Hargreave, F. 1990. "Outpatient Management of Bronchial Asthma." *Medical Clinics of North America* 74(3):797–809.

Coe, R. 1997. "The Magic of Science and the Science of Magic: An Essay on the Process of Healing." *Journal of Health and Social Behavior* 38:1–8.

Cohen, L. 1987. "Bibliotherapy: Using Literature to Help Children

Deal with Difficult Problems." *Journal of Psychosocial Nursing and Mental Health Services* 25(10):20−24.

Cohen, M., Gur, E., Wertheym, E., and Shafir, R. 1995. "Intranasal Administration of Midazolam with a Dinosaur Toy." *Plastic and Reconstructive Surgery* 95(2):421−422.

Cohen, T. 1999. *Jokes: Philosophical Thoughts on Joking Matters.* Chicago: University of Chicago Press.

Cohen. L. and Panopoulos, G. 1997. "Nurse Coaching and Cartoon Distraction: An Effective and Practical Intervention to Reduce Child, Parent, and Nurse Distress During Immunizations." *Journal of Pediatric Psychology* 22(3):355−370.

Cole, R. and. Reiss, D. (eds.) 1993. *How Do Families Cope With Chronic Illness?* Hillsdale, NJ: Lawrence Erlbaum.

Corsaro, W. and Miller, P. J. (eds.) 1992. *Interpretive Approaches to Children's Socialization.* San Francisco: Jossey-Bass.

Coser, R. 1959. "Some Social Functions of Laughter: A Study of Humor in a Hospital Setting." *Human Relations* 12:171−182.

Cox, B. and Lightfoot, C. (eds.) 1997. *Sociogenetic Perspectives on Internalization.* Mahwah, NJ: Lawrence Erlbaum.

Creer, T. and Burns, K. 1978. "Self-Management Training for Children with Chronic Bronchial Asthma." *Psychotherapy and Psychosomatics* 32:270−278.

Creer, T., Stein, R., Rappaport, L., and Lewis, C. 1992. "Behavioral Consequences of Illness: Childhood Asthma as a Model." *Pediatrics* 90(5):808−815.

Csordas, T. 1983. "The Rhetoric of Transformation in Ritual Healing." *Culture, Medicine and Psychiatry* 7:333−375.

D'Antonio, I. 1988. "Therapeutic Use of Play in Hospitals." *Nursing Clinics of North America* 19(2):351−359.

Davis, M. and Wallbridge, D. 1981. *Boundary and Space: An Introduction to the Work of D.W. Winnicott.* New York: Brunner/Mazel Publishers.

Deskin, G. and Steckler, G. 1996. *When Nothing Makes Sense: Disaster, Crisis, and Their Effects on Children.* Minneapolis, MN: Fairview Press.

Doak, S. and Wallace, N. 1986. "The Doctors Wear Pajamas." In *Child Life: an Overview* edited by Association for the Care of Children's Health. Washington, DC: Association for the Care of Children's Health.

Donnelly, E. 1994. "Parents of Children with Asthma: An Examination of Family Hardiness, Family Stressors, and Family Functioning." *Journal of Pediatric Nursing* 9(6):398–407.

Dow, J. 1986. "Universal Aspects of Symbolic Healing: A Theoretical Synthesis." *American Anthropologist* 88:56–69.

Drash, A. and Berlin, N. 1985. "Juvenile Diabetes." In *Issues in the Care of Children with Chronic Illness: A Sourcebook on Problems, Services, and Policies*, edited by N. Berlin and J. Perrin. San Francisco: Jossey-Bass.

Dundes, A. 1987. "At Ease, Disease—AIDS Jokes as Sick Humor." *American Behavior Scientist* 30(1).

Early, E. 1994. *The Raven's Return: The Influence of Psychological Trauma on Individuals and Culture.* Wilmette, IL: Chiron.

Edwards, R. and Alldred, P. 1999. "Children and Young People's Views of Social Research: The Case of Research on Home-School Relations." *Childhood* 6(2):261–281.

Eiser, C. 1990. *Chronic Childhood Disease: An Introduction to Psychological Theory and Research.* Cambridge, UK: Cambridge University Press.

Erikson, E. 1950. *Childhood and Society.* New York: Norton.

Erkolahti, R. 1991. "Transitional Objects and Children with Chronic Disease." *Psychotherapy and Psychosomatics* 56:94–97.

Evaldsson, A. and Corsaro, W. 1998. "Play and Games in the Peer Cultures of Preschool and Preadolescent Children: An Interpretive Approach." *Childhood* 5(4):377–402.

Fanurik, D., Koh, J. L., and Schmitz, M. L. 2000. "Distraction Techniques Combined with EMLA: Effects of IV Insertion Pain and Distress In Children." *Children's Health Care* 29(2):87–101.

Fernandez, J. 1986. *Persuasions and Performances: The Play of Tropes in Culture.* Bloomington, IN: Indiana University Press.

Fernandez, J. (ed.) 1991. *Beyond Metaphor: The Theory of Tropes in Anthropology.* Stanford: Stanford University Press.

Fine, G. A. 1979. "Small Groups and Culture Creation: The Idioculture of Little League Baseball Teams." *American Sociological Review* 44:733–745.

Fine, G. A. 1984. "Humorous Interaction and the Social Construction of Meaning." *Studies in Symbolic Interaction* 5:83–101.

Folkman, S. and Moskowitz, J. 2000. "Positive Affect and the Other Side of Coping." *American Psychologist* 55(6):647–654.

Fosson, A. and Husband, E. 1984. "Bibliotherapy for Hospitalized Children." *Southern Medical Journal* 77(3):342–346.

Frank, A. 1995. *The Wounded Storyteller.* Chicago: University of Chicago Press.

Frankenfield, P. 1996. "The Power of Humor and Play as Nursing Interventions for a Child with Cancer: A Case Report." *Journal of Pediatric Oncology Nursing* 13(1):15–20.

Freeman, J., Epston, D., and Lobovits, D. 1997. *Playful Approaches to Serious Problems: Narrative Therapy with Children and Their Families.* New York: Norton.

Freud, S. 1916. *Wit and Its Relation to the Unconscious.* New York: Dover.

Fritz, G., Rubenstein, S., and Lewiston, N. 1987. "Psychological Factors in Fatal Childhood Asthma." *American Journal of Orthopsychiatry* 57(2):253–257.

Garmezy, N. and Rutter, M. (eds.) 1988. *Stress, Coping and Development in Children.* Baltimore: Johns Hopkins University Press.

Garrison, W. and McQuiston, S. 1989. *Chronic Illness during Childhood and Adolescence: Psychological Aspects.* Newbury Park, CA: Sage.

Gaskins, S. 1996. "How Mayan Parental Theories Come Into Play." In *Parents' Cultural Belief Systems: Their Origins, Expressions, and Consequences,* edited by C. Super and S. Harkness. New York: Guilford.

Gerber, T. A. 1986. "A Secret Vice: A Study of Private Language and Imaginary Kingdoms in Childhood and Adolescence." *Child and Adolescent Social Work* 3(3):151–160.

Gergen, P., Fowler, J., and Maurer, K. 1998. *The Burden of Environmental Tobacco Smoke on the Respiratory Health of Children 2 Months through 5 Years of Age in the United States* [Pediatrics Electronic Pages 101 (2)]. AHCPR Publications Clearinghouse. *http:// www.pediatrics.org.*

Gill, G. 1991. "Psychological Aspects of Diabetes." *British Journal of Hospital Medicine* 46:301–305.

Goffman, E. 1961. *Asylums: Essays on the Social Situation of Mental Patients and Other Inmates.* Garden City, NY: Anchor Books.

Goffman, E. 1963. *Stigma.* New York: Touchstone Press.

Goldman, L. and Smith, C. 1998. "Imagining Identities: Mimetic Constructions in Huli Child Fantasy Play." *Journal of the Royal Anthropological Institute* 4(2):207–234.

Goncu, A., Tuermer, J., Jyoti, J., and Johnson, J. 1999. "Children's Play as Cultural Activity." In *Children's Engagement in the World: Sociocultural Perspectives,* edited by A. Goncu. Cambridge, UK: Cambridge University Press.

Goncu, A. and Gaskins, S. 1998. "The Role of Pretense and Language in the Development of Self." *Human Development* 41(3):200–204.

Good, B. 1994. *Medicine, Rationality, and Experience: An Anthropological Perspective.* Cambridge, UK: Cambridge University Press.

Gorfinkle, K. 1997. *Soothing Your Child's Pain.* Chicago: Contemporary Books.

Gortmacher, S. L. 1985. "Demography of Chronic Childhood Diseases." In *Issues in the Care of Children with Chronic Illness: A Sourcebook on Problems, Services, and Policies,* edited by N. Hobbs and J. Perrin. San Francisco: Jossey-Bass.

Grey, M., Cameron, M., and Thurber, F. 1991. "Coping and Adaptation in Children with Diabetes." *Nursing Research* 40(3):144–149.

Grey, M., Genel, M., and Tamborlane, W. 1980. "Psychosocial Adjustment of Latency-Aged Diabetics: Determinants and Relationship to Control." *Pediatrics* 65:69–73.

Groch, A. 1974. "Jokes and Appreciation of Humor in Nursery School Children." *Child Development* 45:1098–1102.

Haggerty, R., Sherrod, L., Garmezy, N., and Rutter, M. 1996. *Stress,*

Risk, and Resilience in Children And Adolescents. Cambridge, UK: Cambridge University Press.

Haight, W., Wang, X., Fung, H., Williams, K., and Mintz, J. 1999. "Universal, Developmental, and Variable Aspects of Young Children's Play: A Cross-Cultural Comparison of Pretending At Home." *Child Development* 70(6):1477–1488.

Haight, W. and Miller, P. 1993. *Pretending At Home: Early Development in a Sociocultural Context.* Albany, NY: State University of New York Press.

Halterman, J. S., Aligne, C. A., Auinger, P., McBride, J. T., and Szilagyi, P. G. 2000. Inadequate therapy for asthma among children in the United States. *Pediatrics* 105:272–276.

Handelman, D. 1977. "Play and Ritual: Complementary Frames of Meta-Communication." In *It's a Funny Thing, Humor,* edited by Chapman, A. and Foot, H. Oxford: Pergamon Press.

Hausner, R. 1986. "Medication and Transitional Phenomena." *International Journal of Psychoanalytic Psychotherapy* 11:375–398.

Herman, J. 1997. *Trauma and Recovery.* New York: Basic Books.

Hirsch, M. 1994. "The Body as Transitional Object." *Psychotherapy and Psychosomatics* 62:78–81.

Hobbs, N., Perrin, J., and Ireys, H. 1985. *Chronically Ill Children and Their Families.* San Francisco: Jossey-Bass.

Holland, D., Lachiotte, W., Skinner, D., and Cain, C. 1998. *Identity and Agency in Cultural Worlds.* Cambridge, MA: Harvard University Press.

Honig, A. S. 1988. "Humor Development in Children." *Young Children* May, 60–73.

Hubble, M., Duncan, B., and Miller, S. 1999. *The Heart and Soul of Change.* Washington, DC: American Psychological Association.

Hughes, D., McLeod, M., Garner, B., and Goldbloom, R. 1991. "Controlled Trial of a Home and Ambulatory Program for Asthmatic Children." *Pediatrics* 87:54–61.

Hunt, L. and Mattingly, C. 1998. "Diverse Rationalities and Multiple Realities in Illness and Healing." *Medical Anthropology Quarterly* 12(3):267–272.

Hyland, M. E., Kenyon, C.A.P., Allen, R., and Howarth, P. 1993. "Diary Keeping in Asthma: Comparison of Written and Electronic Methods." *British Medical Journal* 306:487–489.

Hymovich, D. and Hagopian, G. 1992. *Chronic Illness in Children and Adults: A Psychosocial Approach.* Philadelphia: W. B. Saunders.

Imber-Black, E., Roberts, J., and Whiting, R. (eds.) 1988. *Rituals in Family and Family Therapy.* New York: Norton Press.

Jacoby, S. and Ochs, E. 1995. "Co-Construction: An Introduction." *Research on Language and Social Interaction.* 28(3):171–184.

James, A. and Prout, A. (eds.) 1997. *Constructing and Reconstructing Childhood.* London: Falmer Press.

Janoff-Bulman, R. 1992. *Shattered Assumptions: Towards a New Psychology of Trauma.* New York: Free Press.

Johnson, M., Whitt, J., and Martin, B. 1987. "The Effect of Fantasy Facilitation of Anxiety in Chronically Ill and Healthy Children." *Journal of Pediatric Psychology* 12(2):273–284.

Johnson, M. T. 1994. "The Doll Clinic: A Preschooler's Guide to Less Fearful Health Care." *Journal of Pediatric Health Care* 8:291–292.

Johnson, S. B., Tomer, A., Cunningham, W., and Henretta, J. 1990. "Adherence in Childhood Diabetes: Results of a Confirmatory Factor Analysis." *Health Psychology* 9(4):493–501.

Judd, D. 1995. *Give Sorrow Words: Working With A Dying Child.* New York: The Haworth Press.

Kampfner, C. 1995. Post-Traumatic Stress Reactions in Children of Imprisoned Mothers." In *Children of Incarcerated Parents,* edited by K. Gabel and D. Jonston. New York: Lexington Books.

Kaplan, E. B. 2000. "Food as a Metaphor for Care." *Journal of Contemporary Ethnography* 29(4):474–509.

Kenderdine, M. 1932. "Laughter in the Pre-School Child." *Child Development* 3:114–136.

Kibirige, M. S. 1993. "Children also Misinterpret the Signs." *British Medical Journal* 307:1210.

Kleiber, C. and Harper, D. 1999. "Effects of Distraction on Children's Pain and Distress during Medical Procedures: A Meta-Analysis." *Nursing Research* 48(1):44–49.

Kleinman, A. 1980. *Patients and Healers in the Context of Culture.* Berkeley: University of California Press.

Kleinman, A. 1988. *The Illness Narratives: Suffering, Healing and the Human Condition.* New York: Basic Books.

Kleinman, A. 1997. " 'Everything That Really Matters': Social Suffering, Subjectivity and the Remaking of Experience in a Disordering World." *The Harvard Theological Review* 90(3):315–335.

Klingelhofer, E. 1987. "Compliance with Medical Regimens, Self-Management Programs, and Self-Care in Childhood Asthma." *Clinical Reviews in Allergy* 5(3):231–247.

Korbin, J. and Zahorik, P. 1985. "Childhood, Health, and Illness: Beliefs and Behaviors of Urban American Schoolchildren." *Medical Anthropology* 9(4):337–353.

Lakoff, G. and Turner, M. 1989. *More Than Cool Reason: A Field Guide to Poetic Metaphor.* Chicago: University of Chicago Press.

Lambert, R. and Lambert, N. 1995. "The Effects of Humor on Secretory Immunoglobulin A Levels in School-Aged Children." *Pediatric Nursing* 21(1):16–19.

Lanphear, B. P., Kahn, R. S., Berger, O., Auinger, P., Bortnick. S. M., and Nahhas, R.W. 2001. "Contribution of Residential Exposures to Asthma in U.S. Children and Adolescents." *Pediatrics* 107(6):E98

Lave, J. and Wenger, E. 1991. *Situated Learning: Legitimate Peripheral Participation.* Cambridge, UK: Cambridge University Press.

Lavigne, J. and Faier-Routman, J. 1992. "Psychological Adjustment to Pediatric Physical Disorders: A Meta-Analytical Review." *Journal of Pediatric Psychology* 17(2):133–157.

Lazarus, R. 1985. "The Costs and Benefits of Denial." In *Stress and Coping: An Anthology,* edited by A. Monat and P. Lazarus. New York: Columbia University Press.

Lehman, E., Arnold, B., and Reeves, S. 1995. "Attachments to Blankets, Teddy Bears, and Other Nonsocial Objects: A Child's Perspective." *The Journal of Genetic Psychology* 156(4):443–459.

Lehman, E., Arnold, B., Reeves, S., and Steler, A. 1996. "Maternal Beliefs about Children's Attachments to Soft Objects." *American Journal of Orthopsychiatry* 66(3):427–436.

Levine, J. 1980. "The Clinical Use of Humor in Work with Children." In *Children's Humor,* edited by P. McGhee and A. Chapman. New York: John Wiley and Sons.

Liess, W., Kapellen, T., Siebler, J., Deutscher, J., Raile, K., Dost, A., Meyer K., and Nietzchumann, U. 1998. "Practical Aspects of Managing Preschool Children with Type 1 Diabetes." *Acta Paediatrica Supplement* 425:67–71.

Litt, C. 1986. "Theories of Transitional Object Attachment: An Overview." *International Journal of Behavioral Development* 9(3): 383–399.

Litt, C. 1981."Children's Attachments to Transitional Objects: A Study of Two Pediatric Populations." *American Journal of Orthopsychiatry* 51:131–139.

Lookabaugh, S. and Fu., V. 1992. "Children's Use of Inanimate Transitional Objects in Coping with Hassles." *Journal of Genetic Psychology* 153(1):37–45.

MacLean, W. 1992. "Psychological Adjustment of Children with Asthma: Effects of Illness Severity and Recent Stressful Events." *Journal of Pediatric Psychology* 17(2):159–171.

Malveaux, F., Houlihan, D., and Diamond, E. 1993. "Characteristics of Asthma Mortality and Morbidity in African-Americans." *Journal of Asthma* 30:431–437.

Manne, S., Bakeman, R., Jacobsen, P., and Redd, W. 1993. "Children's Coping During Invasive Medical Procedures." *Behavior Therapy* 24:143–158.

Marcus, H., Mullally, P. and Kitayma, S. 1997. "Selfways: Diversity in Modes of Cultural Participation." In *The Conceptual Self in Context,* edited by U. Neisser and D. Jopling. New York: Cambridge University Press.

Markham, U. 1998. *Childhood Trauma.* Rockport, MA: Element Books.

Martin, R. and Dobbin, J. 1988. "Sense of Humor, Hassles, and Immunoglobulin A: Evidence for Stress Moderating Effect of Humor." *International Journal of Psychiatry in Medicine* 18(2):93–105.

Mason, S., Johnson, M. H., and Woolley, C. 1999. "A Comparison of

Distracters for Controlling Distress in Young Children during Medical Procedures." *Journal of Clinical Psychology in Medical Settings* 6(3):239–248.

McCormick, E. 1990. "On the Rise: Asthma among Children." *Pharmacy Times* 56(4):90–92.

McCubbin, H., Thompson, E., Thompson, A., and McCubbin, M. 1993. "Family Schema, Paradigms, and Paradigm Shifts: Components and Processes of Appraisal in Family Adaptation to Crisis." In *Cognitive Coping, Families and Disability*, edited by A. Turnbull, J. Patterson, S. Behr, D. Murphy, J. Marquis, and M. Blue-Banning. Baltimore: Paul H. Brookes Publishing.

McCue, K. 1988. "Medical Play: An Expanded Perspective." *Children's Health Care* 16(3):157–161.

McGhee, P. 1989. *Humor and Children's Development.* New York: The Haworth Press.

McGhee, P. 1996. *Health, Healing and the Amuse System.* Dubuque, Iowa: Kendall Hunt Publishing.

McGhee, P. and Johnson, S. 1975. "The Role of Fantasy and Reality Cues In Children's Appreciation of Incongruity Humor." *Merrill Palmer Quarterly* 21(1):19–30.

Mechling, J. 1995. "Children's Folklore in Residential Institutions." In Sutton- *Children's Folklore: A Sourcebook*, edited by B. Smith, J. Mechling, T. Johnson, and F. McMahon. New York: Garland Publishing.

Meza, C. and Gershwin, M. 1997. "Why Is Asthma Becoming More of a Problem? "*Current Opinion in Pulmonary Medicine* 3(1):6–9.

Miller, B. and Strunk, R. 1989. "Circumstances Surrounding the Deaths of Children Due To Asthma: A Case-Control Study." *American Journal of the Diseases of Children* 143:1294 -1299.

Miller, B. and Wood, B. 1991. "Childhood Asthma in Interaction with Family, School, and Peer Systems: A Developmental Model for Primary Care." *Journal of Asthma* 28(6):405–414.

Miller, J. 1988. "Jokes and Joking: A Serious Laughing Matter." In *Laughing Matters: A Serious Look at Humor,* edited by J. Durant and J. Miller. Essex, England: Longman.

Miller, P. 1994. "Narrative Practices: Their Role in Socialization and Self-Construction." In *The Remembering Self: Construction and Accuracy in the Self Narrative,* edited by U. Neisser and R. Fivush. New York: Cambridge University Press.

Miller, P. and Goodnow, J. 1995. "Cultural Practices: Toward an Integration of Culture and Development." In *Cultural Practices as Contexts for Development,* edited by J. Goodnow, P. Miller, and F. Kessel. San Francisco: Jossey-Bass.

Miller, P., Hoogstra, L., Mintz, J., Fung, H., and Williams, K. 1993. "Troubles In The Garden and How They Get Resolved: A Young Child's Transformation of His Favorite Story." In *Memory and Affect in Development,* edited by C. Nelson. Hillsdale, NJ: Lawrence Earlbaum.

Miller, P., Mintz, J., Hoogstra, L., Fung, H., and Potts, R. 1992. "The Narrated Self: Young Children's Construction of Self In Relation To Others in Conversational Stories of Personal Experience." *Merrill-Palmer Quarterly* 38:45–67.

Miller, P., Potts, R., Fung, H., Hoogstra, L., and Mintz, J. 1990. "Narrative Practices and the Social Construction of Self in Childhood." *American Ethnologist* 17:292–311.

Miller, P., Wiley, A., Fung, H., and Liang, C. 1997. "Personal Storytelling as a Medium of Socialization In Chinese and American Families." *Child Development* 68:557–568.

Miller, T. (ed.) 1998. *Children of Trauma: Stressful Life Events and Their Effects on Children and Adolescents.* Madison, CT: International Universities Press.

Mindess, H. 1987. "The Panorama of Humor and the Meaning of Life." *American Behavior Scientist* 30(1):82–95.

Mintz, L. 1985. "Stand-up Comedy as Social and Cultural Mediation." *American Quarterly* 37(1):71–80.

Monahon, C. 1993. *Children and Trauma: A Parents Guide to Helping Children Heal.* New York: Lexington Books.

Monat, A. and Lazarus, R. 1985. *Stress and Coping: An Anthology.* New York: Columbia University Press.

Monighan-Nourot, P., Scales, B., Hoorn, J. V., and Almy, M. 1987. *Looking At Children's Play: A Bridge between Theory and Practice.* New York: Teacher's College Press.

Morgan, W. and Martinez, F. 1992. "Risk Factors for Developing Wheezing and Asthma In Childhood." *Pediatric Clinics of North America* 39(6):1185–1203.

Morris, D. 1997. "Placebo, Pain and Belief: A Biocultural Model." In *The Placebo Effect: An Interdisciplinary Exploration,* edited by A. Harrington. Cambridge, MA: Harvard University Press.

Murphy, R. 1987. *The Body Silent.* New York: W.W. Norton.

Nemeroff, C. and Rozin, P. 1989. "'You are what you eat' Applying the demand-free "impressions" technique to an unacknowledged belief." *Ethos* 17:50–69.

Olsen, B., Sjolie, A., Hougaard, P., Johannesen, J., Borch-Johnsen, K., Marinelli, K., Thorsteinsson, B., Pramming, S., Mortensen, H., and the Danish Study Group of Diabetes in Childhood 2000. "A 6-Year Nationwide Cohort Study of Glycaemic Control In Young People with Type 1 Diabetes: Risk Markers For The Development of Retinopathy, Nephropathy, and Neuropathy." *Journal of Diabetes and Its Complications* 14(6):295–300.

Oremland, E. 2000. *Protecting the Emotional Development of the Ill Child: The Essence Of The Child Life Profession.* Madison, CT: Psychosocial Press.

Ory, M. and Kronenfeld, J. 1980. "Living with Juvenile Diabetes Mellitus." *Pediatric Nursing* 6(5):47–50.

Pardeck, J. and Pardeck, J. 1993. *Bibliotherapy: A Clinical Approach for Helping Children.* Yverdon, Switzerland: Gordon and Breach Science Publishers.

Parikh, N. and Schneider, M. 1988. Book Buddies: Bringing Stories to Hospitalized Children. *School Library Journal* 35:35–39.

Patrice, M. 1993. *Ritual: Power, Healing and Community.* New York: Penguin Books.

Patterson, J. 1993. "The Role of Family Meanings in Adaptation to Chronic Illness and Disability." In *Cognitive Coping, Families and Disability,* edited by A. Turnbull, J. Patterson, S. Behr, D. Murphy, J. Marquis, M. Blue-Banning. Baltimore: Paul H. Brookes Publishing.

Pendleton, S., Cavalli, B., Pargament, K., and Nasr, S. 2002. "Religious/Spiritual Coping in Childhood Cystic Fibrosis: A Qualitative Study." *Pediatrics* 109:1.

Perrin, E. and Gerrity, P. 1984. "Development of Children with a Chronic Illness." *Pediatric Clinics of North America* 31(1).

Perrin, E. and Gerrity, S. 1981. "There's A Demon In Your Belly: Children's Understanding of Illness." *Pediatrics* 67:841–849.

Perrin, E., Sayer, A., and Willett, J. 1991. "Sticks and Stones May Break My Bones . . . Reasoning about Illness Causality and Body Functioning in Children who have a Chronic Illness." *Pediatrics* 88: 608–619.

Perrin, J., MacLean, W., and Perrin, E. 1989. "Parental Perceptions of Health Status and Psychological Adjustment of Children with Asthma." *Pediatrics* 83(1):26–30.

Piaget, J. 1962. *Play, Dreams and Imitation In Childhood.* New York: Norton.

Pillemer, D. 1998. *Momentous Events, Vivid Memories: How Unforgettable Moments Help Us Understand the Meaning of Our Lives.* Cambridge, MA: Harvard University Press.

Plaut, T. 1988. *Children with Asthma: A Manual for Parents.* Amherst, MA: Pedipress.

Potts, R. 1996. "Spirituality and the Experience of Cancer in an African-American Community: Implications for Psychosocial Oncology." *Journal of Psychosocial Oncology* 14:1–19.

Powers, S. W. 1999. "Empirically Supported Treatments in Pediatric Psychology: Procedure-Related Pain." *Journal of Pediatric Psychology* 24(2):131–145.

Pretzlik, U. 1997. *Children Coping with Serious Illness.* Amsterdam, NL: University of Amsterdam.

Prout, A. 1996. "Actor-Network Theory, Technology and Medical Sociology: An Illustrative Analysis of the Metered Dose Inhaler." *Sociology of Health and Illness* 18(2):198–219.

Prout, A., Hayes, L., and Gelder, L. 1997. *Medicines and the Mainte-nance of Ordinariness and the Household Management of Childhood Asthma*. Staffordshire, UK: Report for EU-BIOMED Project.

Rea, H., Sears, M., Beaglehole, R., Fenwick, J., Jackson, R., Gillies, A., O'Donnell, T., Holst, P., and Rothwell, P. 1987. "Lessons from the National Asthma Mortality Study: Circumstances Surrounding Death." *New Zealand Medical Journal* 100:10–13.

Rich, M., Lamola, S., Amory, C., and Schneider, L. 2000. "Asthma in Life Context: Video Intervention/Prevention Assessment." *Pedi-atrics* 105:469–477.

Rich, M. and Chalfen, R. 1999. "Showing and Telling Asthma: Chil-dren Teaching Physicians with Visual Narratives." *Visual Sociology* 14:51–71.

Riordan, R. 1991. "Bibliotherapy Revisited." *Psychological Reports* 68(1):306.

Roberts, J. 1988. "Setting the Frame: Definition, Functions and Typol-ogy of Rituals." In *Rituals In Families and Family Therapies* edited by E. Imber-Black, J. Roberts, and R. Whiting. New York: Norton.

Robinson, V. 1991. *Humor and the Health Professions*. Thorofare, NJ: Slack.

Roopnarine, J., Johnson, J., and Hooper, F. 1994. *Children's Play in Di-verse Cultures*. Albany, NY: State University of New York Press.

Rozin, P. 1990. "The Importance of Social Factors in Understanding the Acquisition of Food Habits." In *Taste, Experience, and Feeding: Development and Learning* edited by E. Capaldi and T. Powley. Washington, DC: American Psychological Association.

Rushforth, H. 1999. "Practitioner Review: Communicating With Hos-pitalized Children: Review and Application of Research Pertaining to Children's Understanding of Health and Illness." *Journal of Child Psychology and Psychiatry* 40(5):683–691.

Ryan-Wenger, N. and Walsh, M. 1994. "Children's Perspectives on Coping with Asthma." *Pediatric Nursing* 20(3):224–228.

Ryden, O., Nevander, L., Johnson, P., Westbom, L., and Sjoblad, S. 1990. "Diabetic Children and Their Parents: Personality Correlates of Metabolic Control." *Acta Paediatrica Scandinavica* 79:1204–1212.

Sander, N. 1994. *A Parent's Guide to Asthma.* New York: Plume Books.

Sarbin, T. 1997. "The Poetics of Identity." *Theory and Psychology* 7(1): 67–82.

Schachter, S. and Wheeler, L. 1962. "Epinephrine, Chrorpromazine, and Amusement." *Journal of Abnormal and Social Psychology* 65(2): 121–128.

Scheff, T. 1977. "The Distancing of Emotion in Ritual." *Current Anthropology* 18(3):483–505.

Scheff, T. 1979. *Catharsis in Healing, Ritual and Drama.* Berkeley: University of California Press.

Shuman, R. 1996. *The Psychology of Chronic Illness.* New York: Basic Books.

Schwartz, R. 1984. "Children with Chronic Asthma: Care by the Generalist and the Specialist." *Pediatric Clinics of North America* 31(1): 87–103.

Sclabassi, S. H. 1973. "Literature as a Therapeutic Tool: A Review of the Literature on Bibliotherapy." *American Journal of Psychotherapy* 27(1):70–77.

Shafii, T. 1986. "The Prevalence and Use of Transitional Objects: A Study of 230 Adolescents. *Journal of the American Academy of Child Psychiatry* 25:805–808.

Shapiro, G. 1992. "Childhood Asthma: An Update." *Pediatrics in Review* 13(11):403–412.

Sherman, L. W. 1975. "An Ecological Study of Glee in Small Groups of Preschool Children." *Child Development* 46:53–61.

Sherman, M., Hertzig, M., Austrian, R., and Shapiro, T. 1981. "Treasured Objects in School-Age Children." *Pediatrics* 68(3):379–386.

Siminerio, L. and Betschart, J. 1986. *Children with Diabetes.* American Diabetes Association.

Singer, D. 1993. *Playing for Their Lives: Helping Troubled Children Through Play Therapy.* New York: Free Press.

Singer, D. 1994. "Play as Healing." In *Toys, Play and Child Development,* edited by J. Goldstein. Cambridge, UK: Cambridge University Press.

Somé, M. P. 1993. *Ritual: Power, Healing and Community.* New York: Penguin Books.

Sourkes, B. 1995. *Armfuls of Time: The Psychological Experience of the Child with Life-Threatening Illness.* Pittsburgh: University of Pittsburgh Press.

Stevenson, O. 1954. "The First Treasured Possession: A Study of the Part Played by Specially Loved Objects and Toys in the Lives of Certain Children." *The Psychoanalytic Study of the Child* 9:199–217.

Strauss, A. 1975. *Chronic Illness and the Quality of Life.* St. Louis: C.V. Mosby Co.

Sutton-Smith, B. 1997. *The Ambiguity of Play.* Cambridge, MA: Harvard University Press.

Taggart, V., Zuckerman, A., Sly, R., Steinmueller, C., Newman, G., O'Brien, R., Schneider, S., and Bellanti, J. 1991. "You Can Control Asthma: Evaluation of an Asthma Education Program for Hospitalized Inner-City Children." *Patient Education and Counseling* 17:35–47.

Taylor, M. 1999. *Imaginary Companions and the Children Who Create Them.* New York: Oxford University Press.

Taylor, S., Aspenwall, L., Giulano, T., Dakoff, G., and Reardon, K. 1993. "Storytelling and Coping with Stressful Events." *Journal of Applied Social Psychology* 23(9):703–733.

Taylor, S., Pham, L., Rivkin, I., and Armor, D. 1998. "Harnessing the Imagination: Mental Simulation, Self-Regulation, and Coping." *American Psychologist* 53(4):429–439.

Taylor, W. and Newacheck, P. 1992. "Impact of Childhood Asthma on Health." *Pediatrics* 90(5):657–662.

Terr, L. 1990. *Too Scared to Cry.* New York: Basic Books.

Thompson, R. J. and Gustafson, K. E. 1996. *Adaptation to Chronic Childhood Illness.* Washington, DC: American Psychological Association.

Turner, V. 1969. *The Ritual Process: Structure and Anti-Structure.* Ithaca: Cornell University Press.

Van Blerkon, L. M. "Clown Doctors: Shamanic Healers of Western Medicine." *Medical Anthropological Quarterly* 9(4):462–475.

Van Der Geest, S. and Whyte, S. R. 1989. The Charm of Medicines: Metaphors and Metonyms." *Medical Anthropological Quarterly* 3(4):345–367.

Van Der Hart, O. 1988. *Rituals in Psychotherapy.* Boston: Houghton-Mifflin.

Van Der Kolk, B., McFarlane, A. and Weisaeth, L. (eds.) 1996. *Traumatic Stress: the Effects of Overwhelming Experience on Mind, Body and Society.* New York: Guilford Press.

Van Deusen, S., Goldin-Meadow, S. and Miller, P. 2001. "Enacting Stories Seeing Worlds: Similarities and Differences in the Cross-Cultural Narrative Development of Linguistically Isolated Children." *Human Development* 44:311–336.

Van Gennep, A. 1960. *The Rites of Passage.* Chicago: University of Chicago Press.

Van Manen, M. 1997. "From Meaning to Method." *Qualitative Health Research* 7(3):345–369.

Vessey, J. A., Carlson, K. L., and McGill, J. 1994. "Use of distraction with children during an acute pain experience." *Nursing Research* 43(6):369–372.

Vygotsky, L.S. 1967. "Play and its Role in the Mental Development of the Child." *Soviet Psychology* 5:6–18.

Walsh, M. and Ryan-Wenger, N. 1992. "Sources of Stress in Children with Asthma." *Journal of School Health* 62(10):459–463.

Ward, D. 1992. "An International Comparison of Asthma Morbidity and Mortality in U.S. Soldiers, 1984 to 1988." *Chest* 101:613–620.

Wartenberg, D., Ehrlich, R. and Lilienfeld, D. 1994. "Environmental Tobacco Smoke and Childhood Asthma: Comparing Exposure Metrics Using Probability Plots." *Environmental Research* 64:122–135.

Webb, N. B. 1991. *Play Therapy with Children in Crisis: A Casebook for Practitioners.* New York: Guilford Press.

Weinstein, A. 1987. *Asthma: The Complete Guide to Self-Management of Asthma and Allergies for Patients and Their Families.* New York: Fawcett Crest.

Wetzman, M., Gortmaker, S., Sobol, A., and Perrin, J. 1992. "Recent Trends in the Prevalence and Severity of Childhood Asthma." *Journal of the American Medical Association* 268(19):2673–2677.

Wiley, A., Rose, A., Burger, L., and Miller, P. 1998. "Constructing Autonomous Selves through Narrative Practices: A Comparative Study of Working-Class and Middle-Class Families." *Child Development* 69:833–847.

Wilkinson, S. 1988. *The Child's World of Illness.* New York: Cambridge University Press.

Wilson, C. 1979. *Jokes: Form, Content, Use and Function.* London: Academic Press.

Wilson, J. 1985. Play in the hospital. In *Play Interactions: The Role of Toys and Parental Involvement in Children's Development,* edited by C. Brown, and A. Gottfried. Skillman, NJ: Johnson and Johnson.

Wilson, S. and Starr-Schneidkraut, N. 1994. "State of the Art in Asthma Education: The U.S. Experience." *Chest* 106(4):197S-205S.

Winnicott, D. W. 1958. "Transitional Objects and Transitional Phenomena." *Collected Papers.* New York: Basic Books.

Wolfenstein, M. 1954. *Children's Humor: A Psychological Analysis.* Glencoe, IL: Free Press.

Wolin, S. and Bennett, L. 1984. "Family Rituals." *Family Process* 23:401–420.

Wooley, J. 1997. "Thinking about Fantasy: Are Children Fundamentally Different Thinkers and Believers from Adults?" *Child Development* 68:208–216.

Wooley, J., Phelps, K., Davis, D., and Mandell, D. 1999. "Where Theories of Mind Meet Magic: The Development of Children's Beliefs about Wishing." *Child Development* 70(3):571–587.

Wooten, P. 1996. *Compassionate Laughter: Jest for Your Health.* Salt Lake City: Commune-A-Key.

Ybarra, G., Passman, P., and Eisenberg, C. 1997. *Security Blanket or Mother: Which Benefits Linus during Pediatric Examinations?* Presented at the American Psychological Association national meeting. Chicago.

Yoos, H. and McMullen, A. 1996. "Illness Narratives of Children with Asthma. *Pediatric Nursing* 22(4):285–290.

Yovetich, N., Dale, A., and Hudak, M. 1990. "Benefits of humor in reduction of threat-induced anxiety." *Psychological Reports* 66:51–58.

Zeltzer, L. and Lebaron, S. 1986. "Fantasy in Children and Adolescents with Chronic Illness." *Developmental and Behavioral Pediatrics* 7(3k20>):195–197.

Index

About the Author

Cindy Dell Clark is on the faculty of Human Development and Family Studies at Penn State Delaware County. She earlier spent nearly two decades as an applied qualitative researcher. In her research today, Clark studies children, culture, and the imagination. She is the author of *Flights of Fancy, Leaps of Faith: Children's Myths in Contemporary America,* in which she explores American childhood rituals such as Santa and the tooth fairy.